EVERYDAY SCIENCE

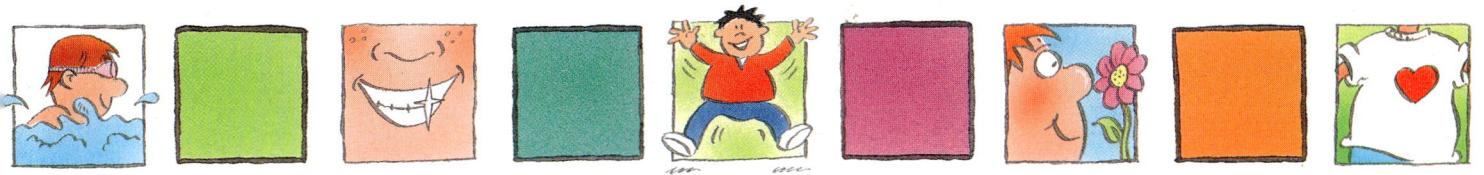

about your body

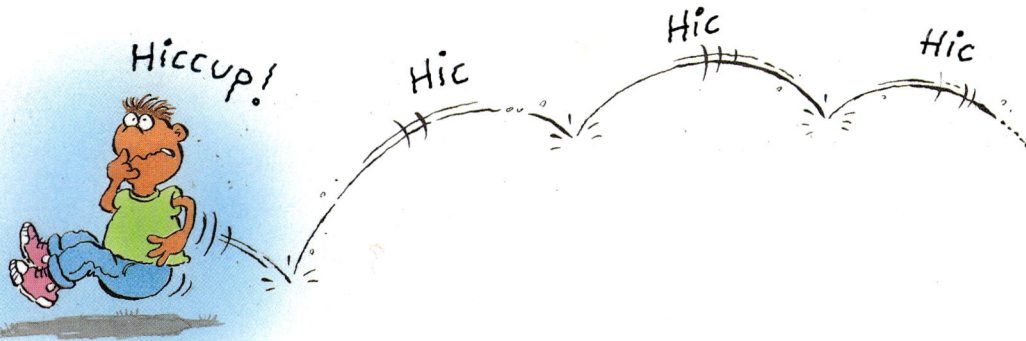

Hiccup! Hic Hic Hic

Barbara Taylor

photography by
Peter Millard

SIMON & SCHUSTER
YOUNG BOOKS

Contents

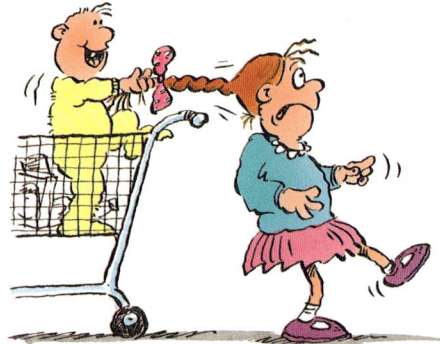

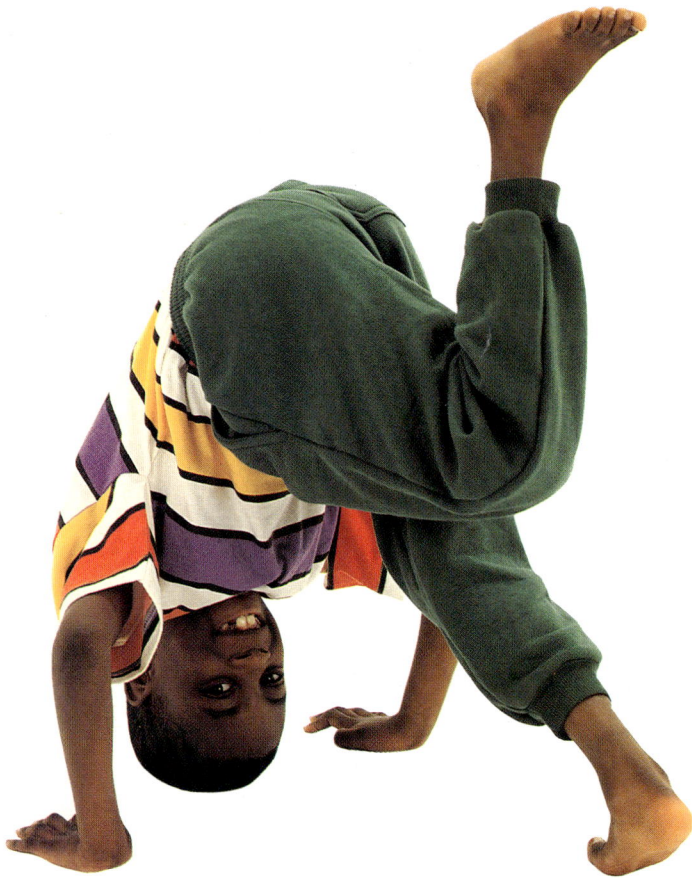

First published in 1994
by Simon & Schuster Young Books

Text © Barbara Taylor 1994
Illustration © Simon & Schuster Young Books 1994

Commissioning editor: Debbie Fox

Illustrators: Joanna Cameron, Simone End,
David Pattison

Design: The Design Works, Reading

The publisher and author would like to thank
Carol Olivier of Kenmont Primary School and the
following children for taking part in the
photography: Farah Bahsoon, Karlene Bellamy,
Kariesha Clarke, Katie Condon, Sandra Gaspar,
Umayema Mahadale, Jay Murfet, Stephen Ousby,
Luke Punter, Kevin Sewell and Saffan Woods.

Thanks also to Elaine Tanner
and the staff of St James' Primary School.

Printed and bound by: Wing King Tong

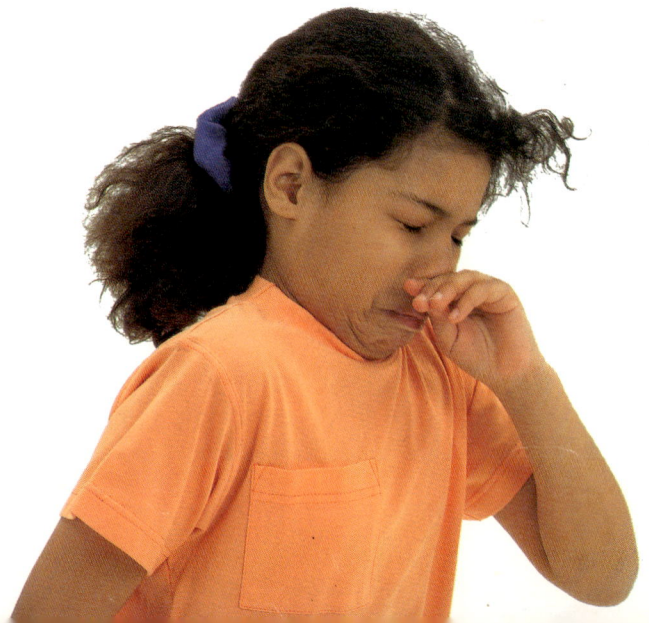

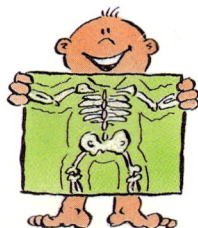

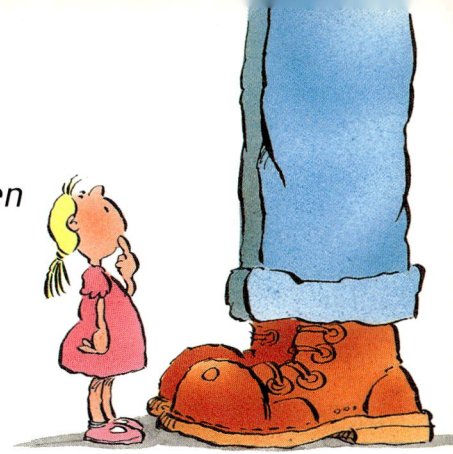

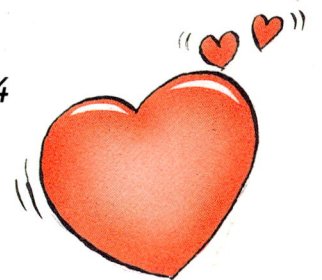

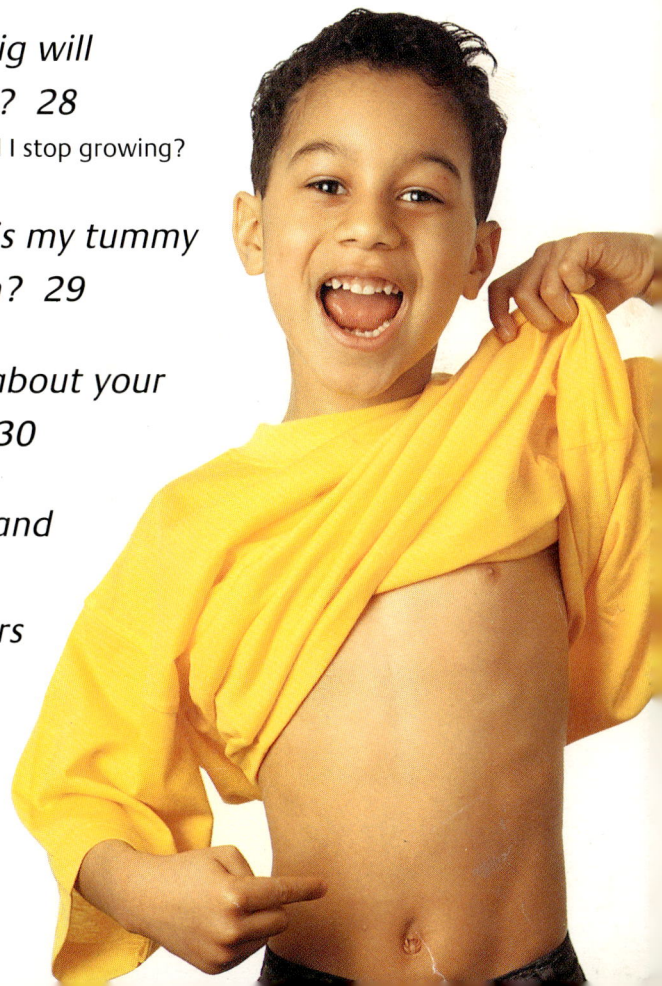

Why is my skin stretchy?

Your skin stretches to give you room to move and grow. It is a watertight bag about 2mm thick which holds your body together.

Your skin is the biggest part of your body.

It stops your insides from drying out and keeps out dirt and germs. It is also sensitive to heat, cold, pressure and pain.

What's under my skin?

Skin is made up of layers. The top layer is dead skin flakes which are rubbed off all the time. Just underneath, new skin grows. The middle layer is made up of living skin. This is where hair and nails start to grow. At the bottom is a layer of fat.

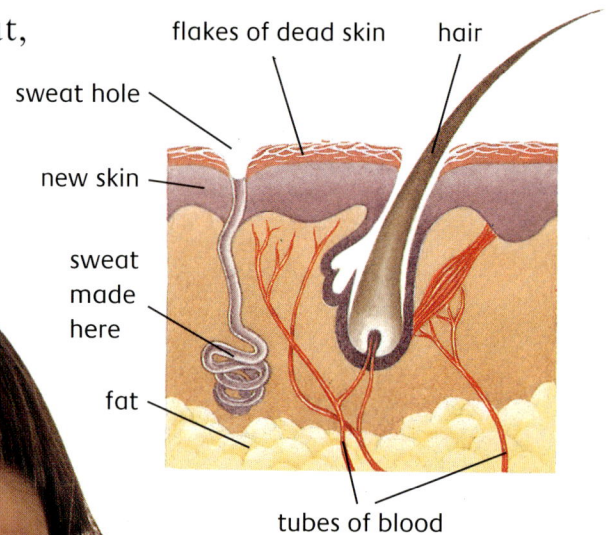

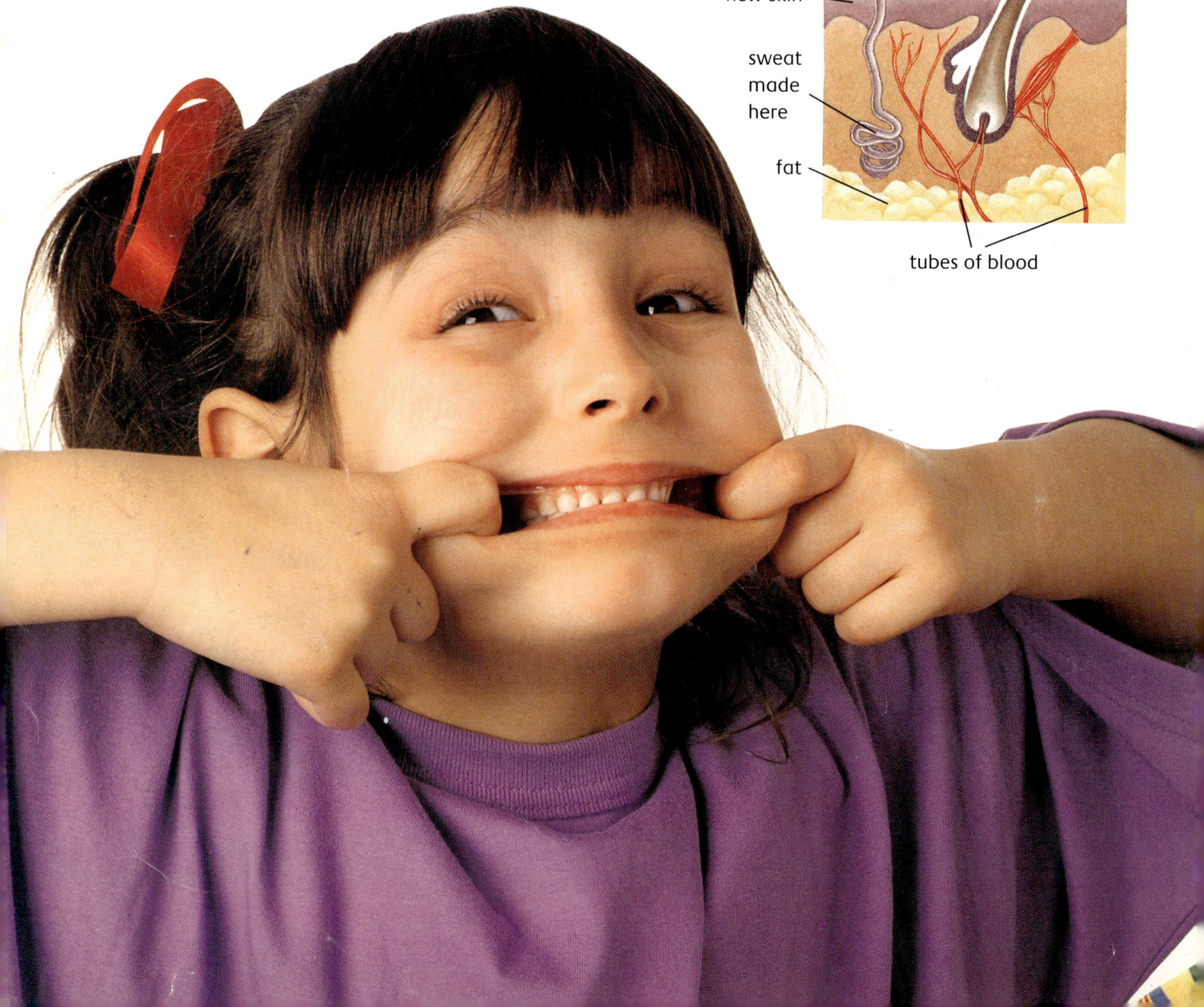

flakes of dead skin

hair

sweat hole

new skin

sweat made here

fat

tubes of blood

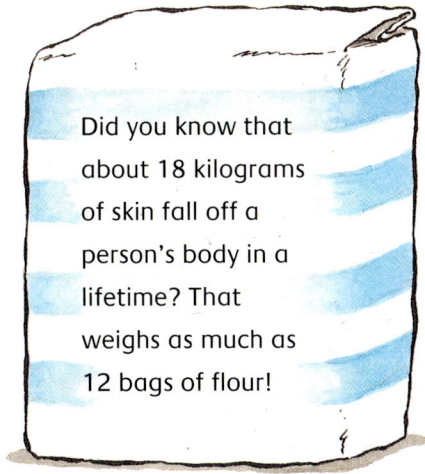

Did you know that about 18 kilograms of skin fall off a person's body in a lifetime? That weighs as much as 12 bags of flour!

Why do I sweat?

When you are hot or scared, sweat comes out of little holes in your skin. Sweat is mostly water and salt. As it dries on the skin, it takes heat away and helps to cool the body down.

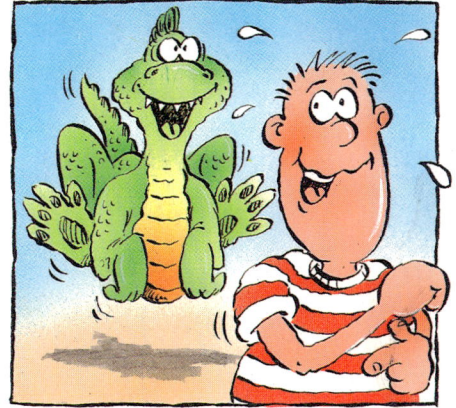

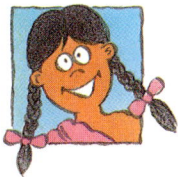

Why do people have different coloured skin?

People with brown or black skin make a lot of coloured dye called melanin in their skin. This helps to protect them from strong, hot sunshine which can hurt or burn the skin. In places with little sun, pale skins are more useful to soak up the sunlight. Some people have little patches of brown melanin called freckles in their skin.

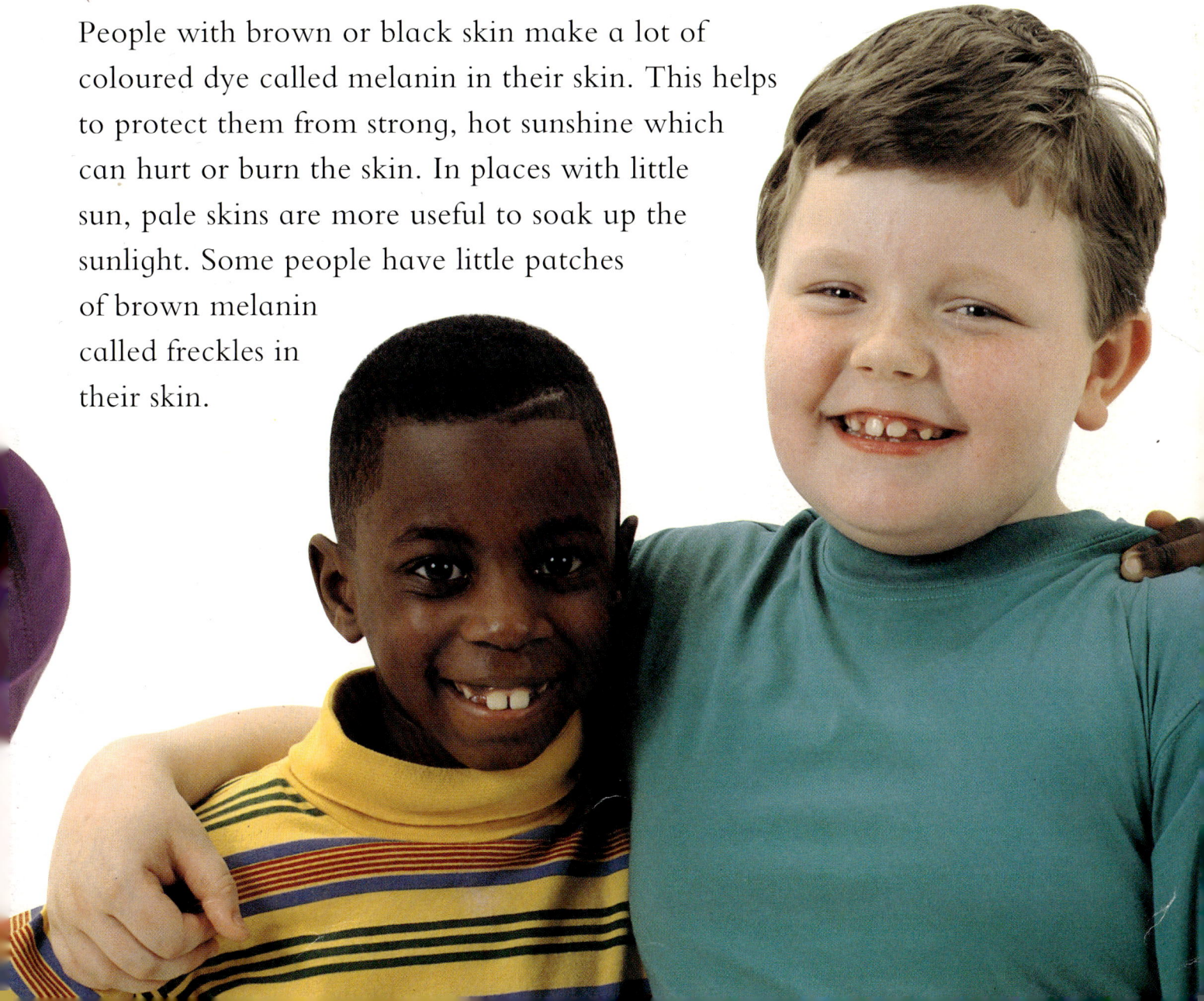

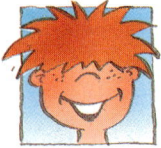

Why am I hairy?

The hair on your head keeps you warm and protects your head from the sun. Eyelashes and eyebrows keep water and dirt out of your eyes and hairs inside your nose and ears trap dust. Years ago, people were much more hairy all over. Their hair helped to keep them warm, like our clothes do today.

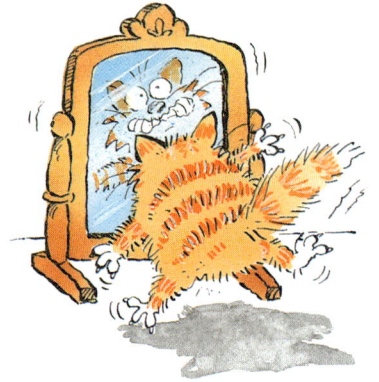

Cats have much more hair than we do. They make their hair stand on end when they are cold or scared. This helps them to keep warm or look fierce.

What are goose pimples?

Goosepimples are one way your body tries to keep warm. Little muscles pull the hair upright, lifting the skin into little bumps. The standing hairs trap a layer of air near the body, which works like a blanket to stop body heat escaping. Unfortunately, people now have so few hairs, this is not a very good way of keeping warm.

Without goosepimples

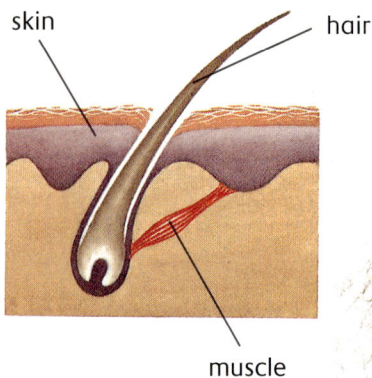

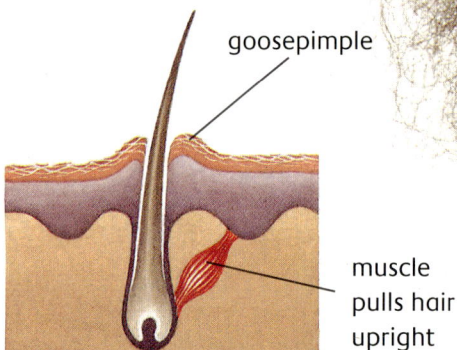

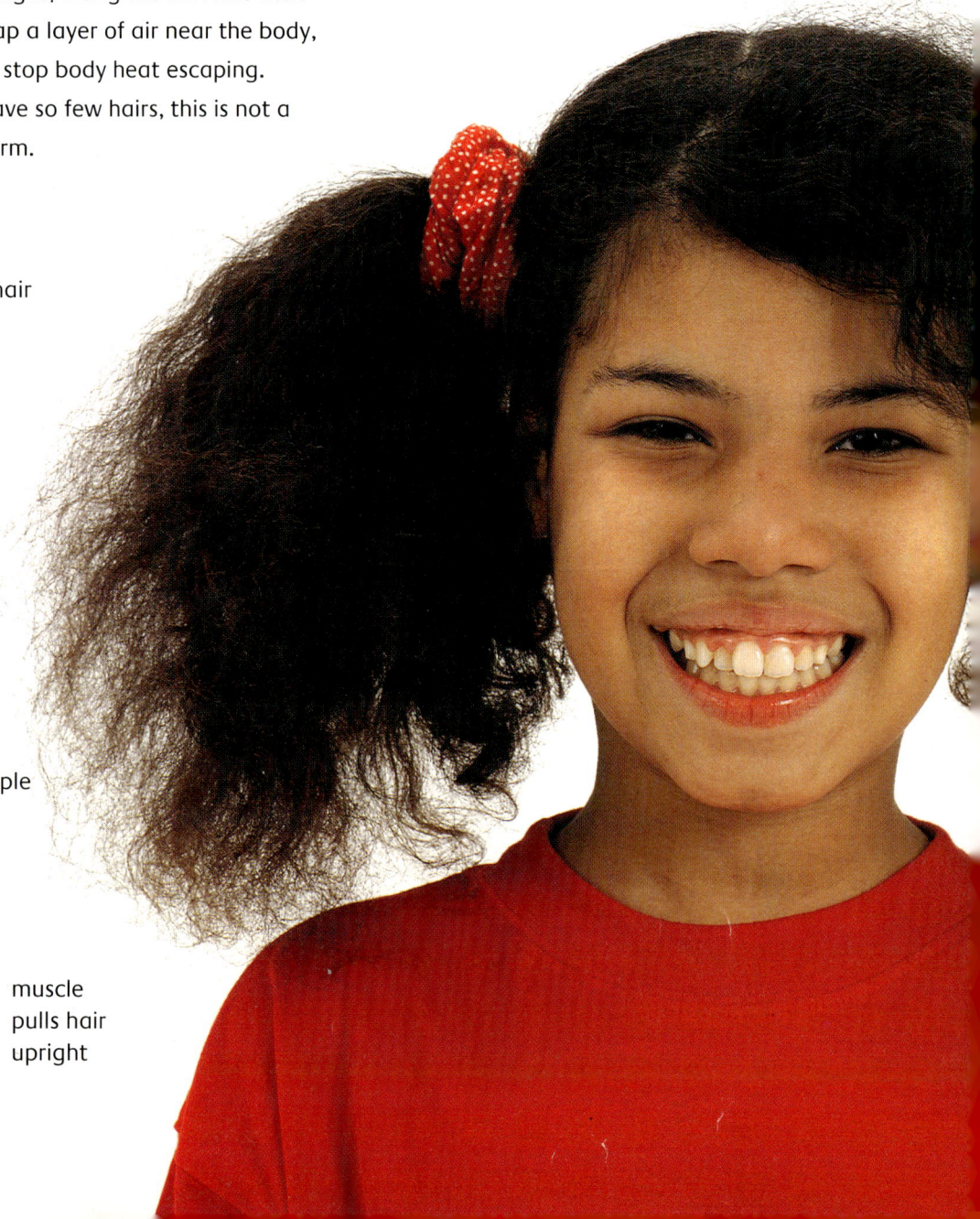

skin   hair

muscle

With goosepimples

goosepimple

muscle pulls hair upright

Why does it hurt when someone pulls my hair?

Although your hair is dead, you can still feel the pain because the roots of your hair are alive.

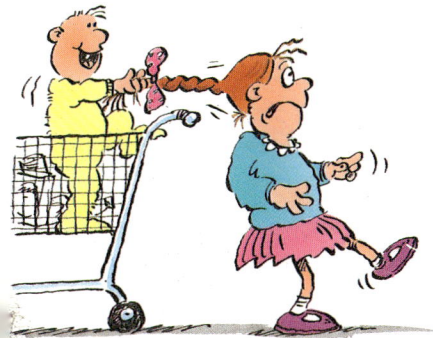

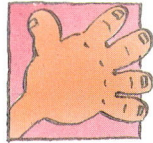

What are my nails for?

Your fingernails and toenails protect the tips of your fingers and toes. They are also useful for picking up little things or for scratching when you itch. Nails are made of the same tough stuff as hair. It is called keratin.

The half moons on your nails look white because the nails are not firmly joined to the skin underneath.

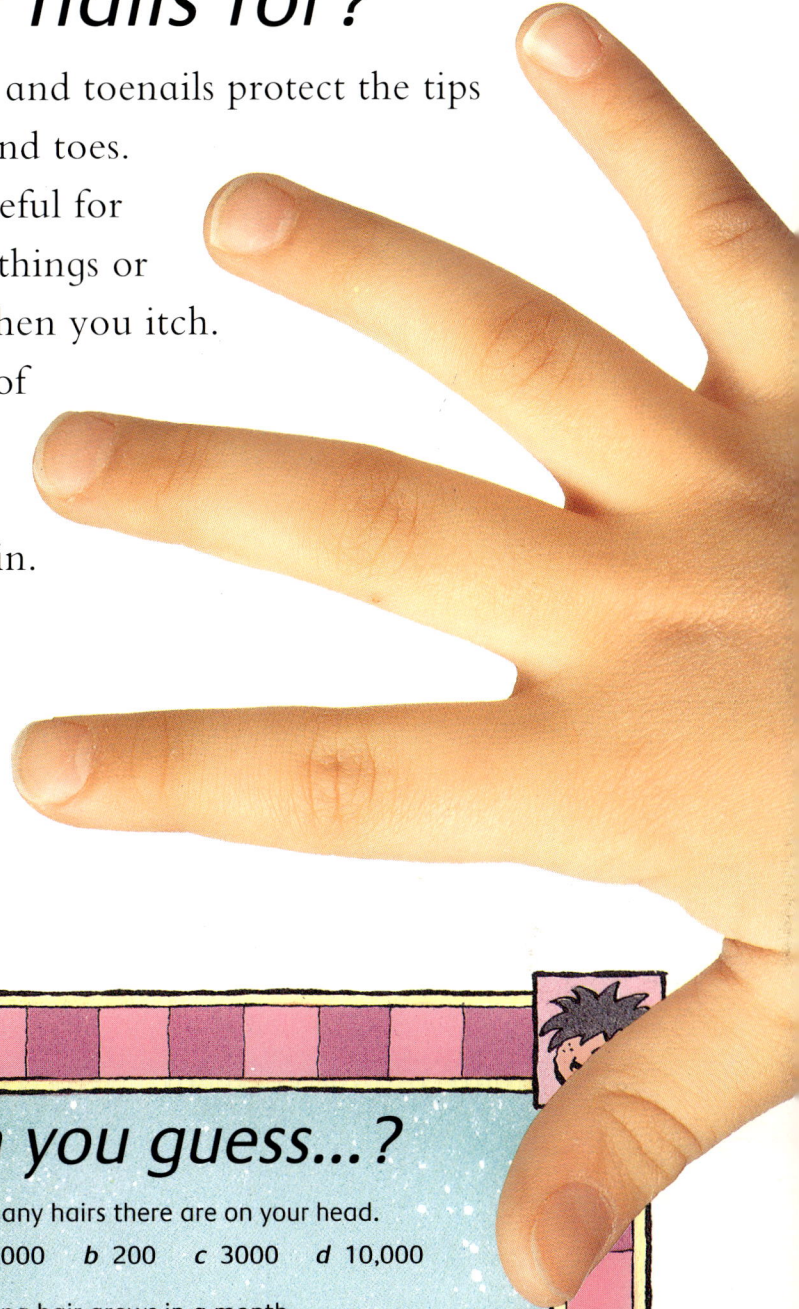

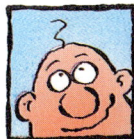

Can you guess...?

1 How many hairs there are on your head.
   a 150,000   b 200   c 3000   d 10,000

2 How long hair grows in a month.
   a 50 mm   b 2 mm   c 10 mm   d 5 mm

3 How long it takes to grow a new fingernail.
   a 1 week   b 1 month   c 3 months   d 6 months

The answers are on page 32.

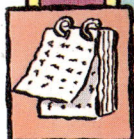

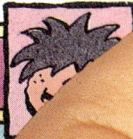

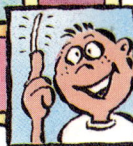

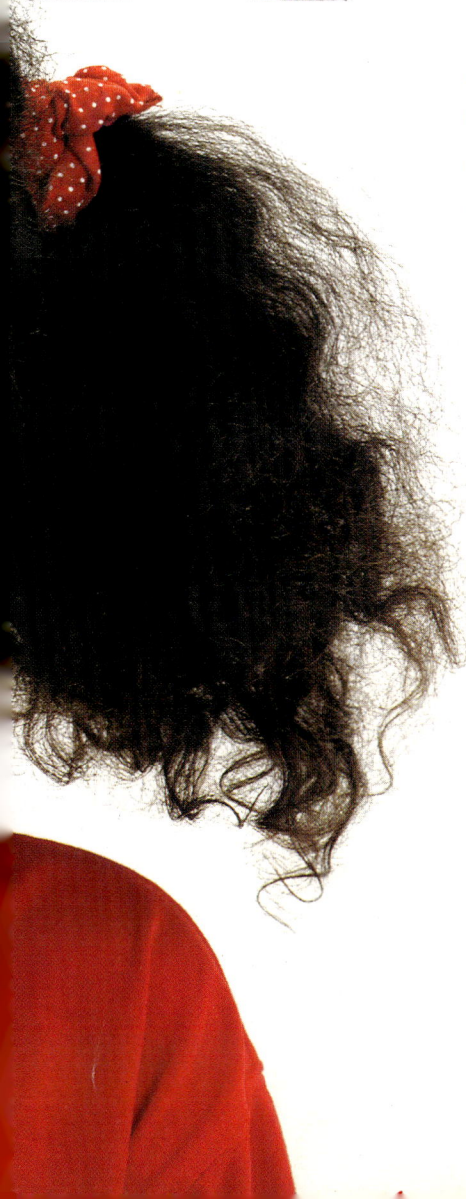

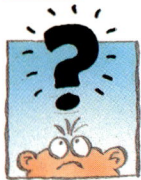

How do I think?

You think with a part of your body called the brain, which is hidden inside your head. Your brain makes thoughts from things you see, hear, feel and remember. When you think, you work out things and make up new ways of doing things. The top part of your brain does most of the thinking.

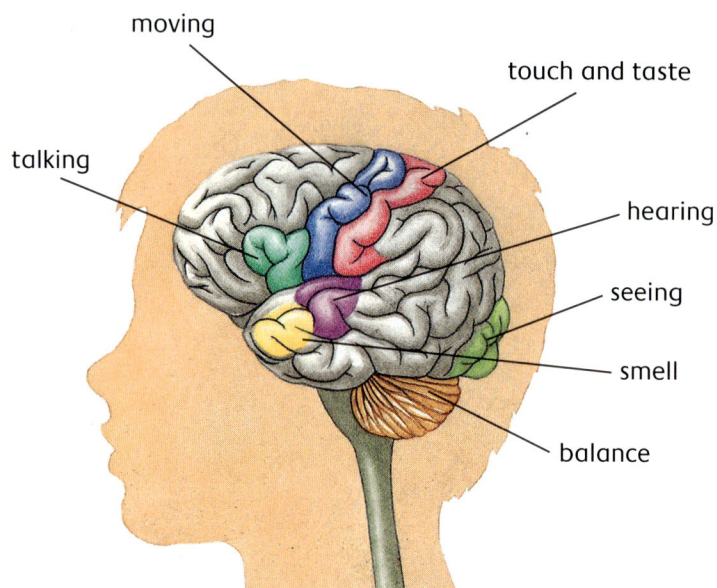

moving

touch and taste

talking

hearing

seeing

smell

balance

What does my brain do?

Different parts of your brain control different things such as seeing, talking or moving. Your brain takes up about half of your head and weighs as much as 13 apples.

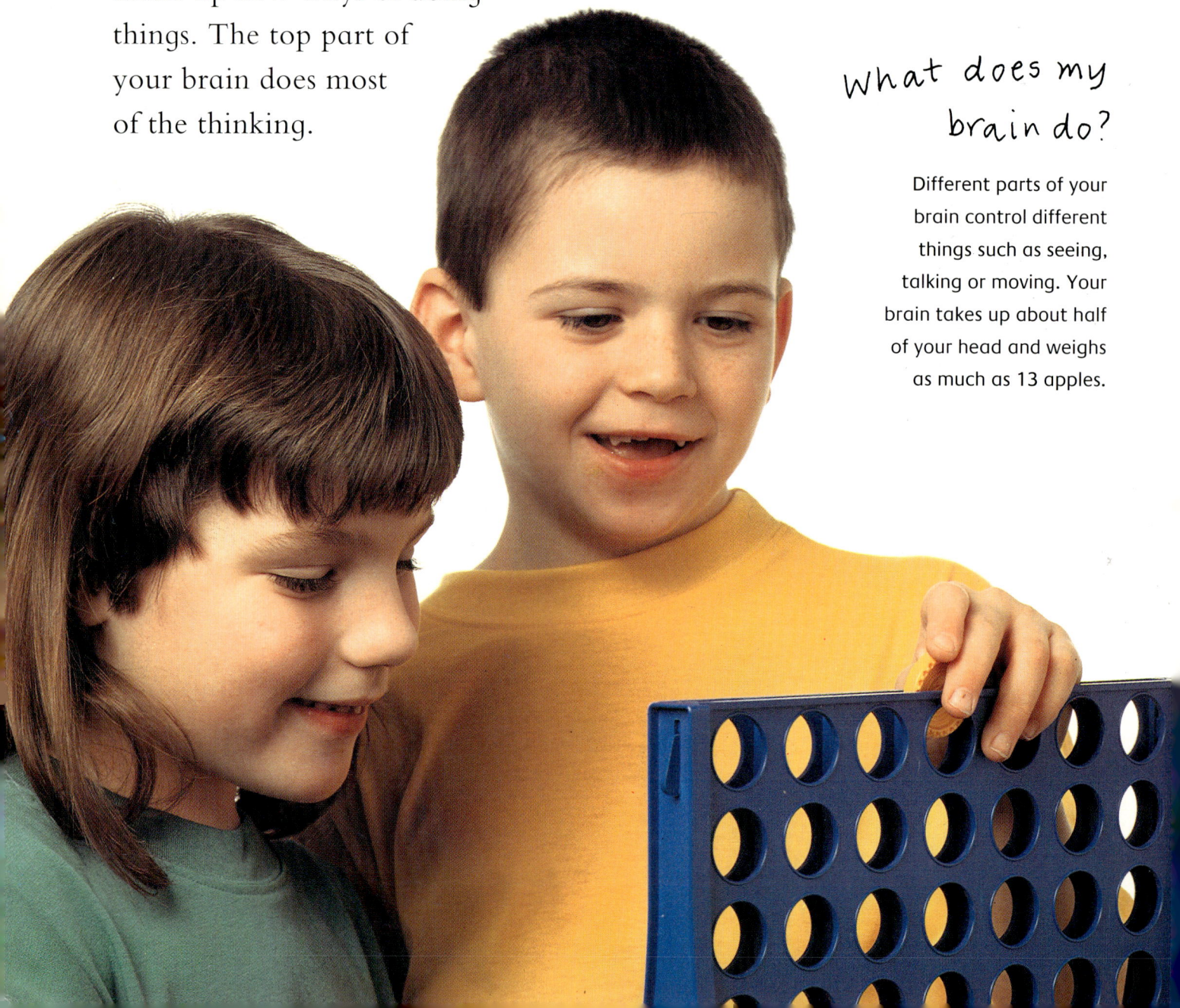

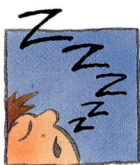

What happens when I sleep?

Your body takes a rest while your brain tries to makes sense of all the things that have happened to you that day. You breathe more slowly, your heart beats more slowly and your muscles relax. You don't hear noises around you.

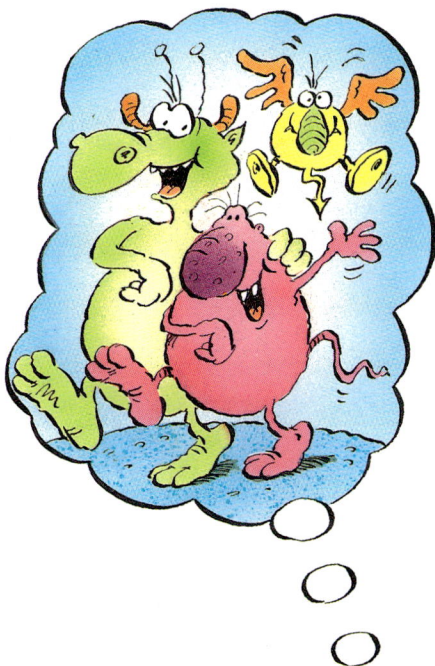

What are dreams?

When you are asleep, your mind floats free and you see pictures in your head – we call this dreaming. Dreams are made up from things you have seen, heard or felt in everyday life. They help you cope with things.

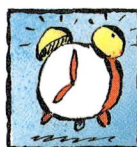

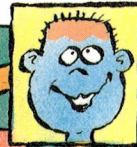

True or false?

1 People sleep for about half their lives.

2 A new-born baby sleeps about 16–20 hours a day.

3 A person's brain is about 80 per cent water.

4 The dinosaur *Stegosaurus* had a brain the size of a small car.

5 Everyone has about five dreams a night.

The answers are on page 32.

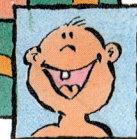

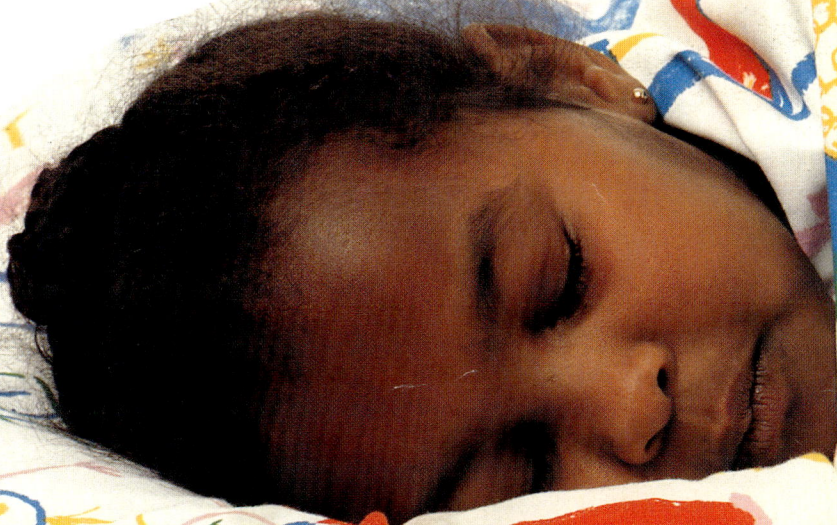

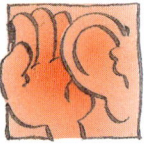

Where does my ear hole go?

Your ear hole leads to a thin circle of skin which is a bit like a drum skin. When sounds in the air hit this eardrum, it shakes. This makes bones and liquids further inside your ear shake as well. They trigger signals which go to your brain and your brain 'hears' the sounds.

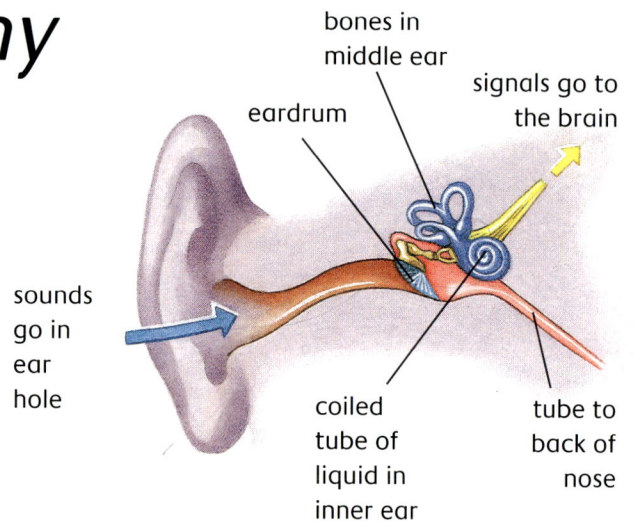

bones in middle ear

signals go to the brain

eardrum

sounds go in ear hole

coiled tube of liquid in inner ear

tube to back of nose

The ear is made up of three main parts. The outer ear, the bit you can see, collects sounds like a funnel. The middle ear inside your head makes the sounds stronger. The inner ear, which is even further inside your head, sends signals to the part of the brain that deals with hearing.

Why are my ears waxy?

The wax in your ears is made by the skin in your ear hole. It traps dirt and dust and carries them out of the ear. The job of ear wax is to keep your ears clean. It is not a good idea to poke anything into your ears.

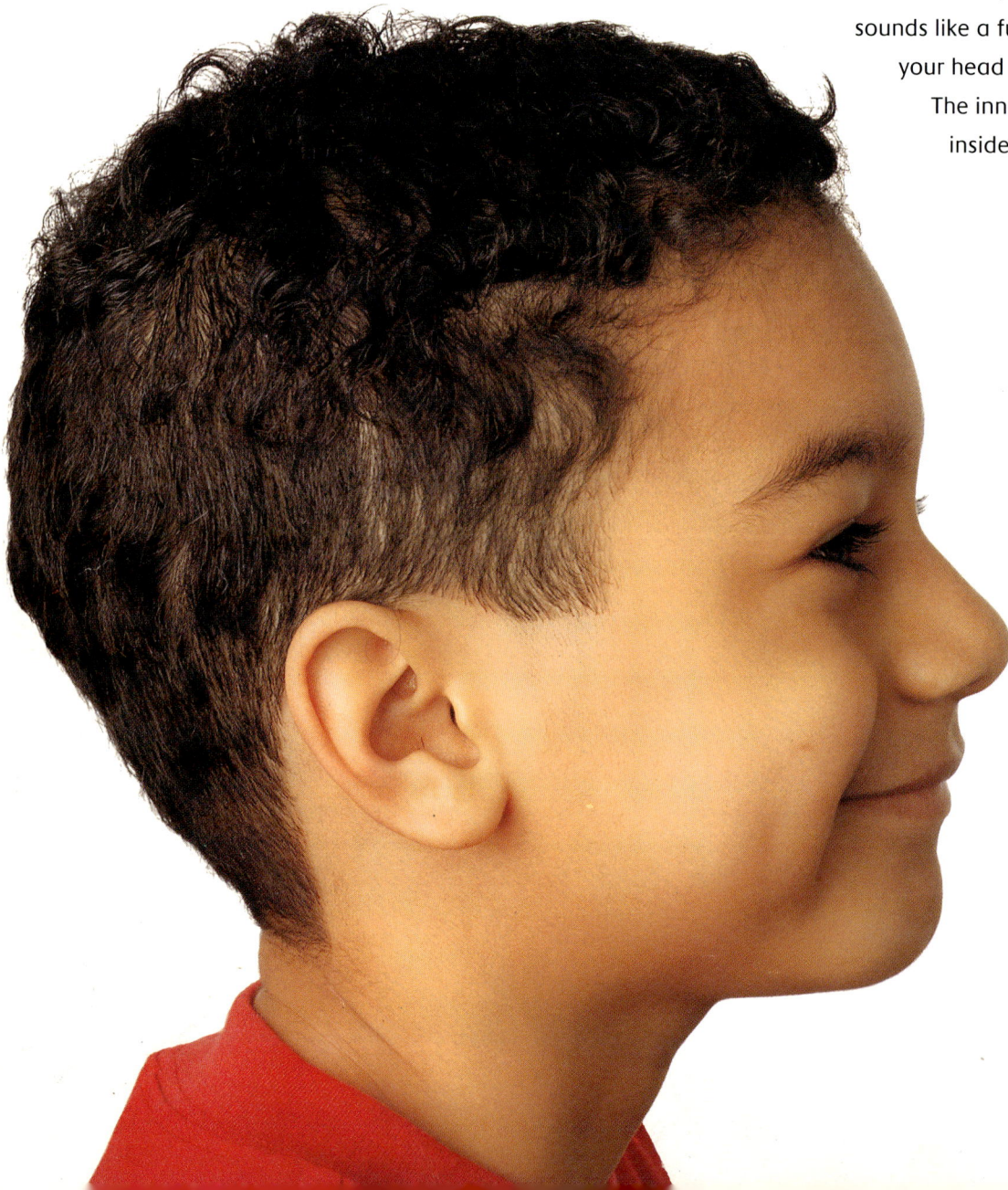

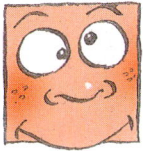

What is the black bit in the middle of my eye?

The black circle is called the pupil. It is really a hole which lets light into your eye. The coloured part of your eye – the iris – makes the pupil bigger or smaller. It controls the amount of light going into your eye. When light goes into your eye, signals go to the back of your brain. The brain sorts out these signals and you see things.

True or false?

1 Cats and dogs cannot see in colour.

2 The salt in tears kills germs and keeps your eyes clean.

3 Crickets have ears on their toes.

4 We have two ears to help us work out which direction a sound is coming from.

5 Tears are made only during the day.

The answers are on page 32.

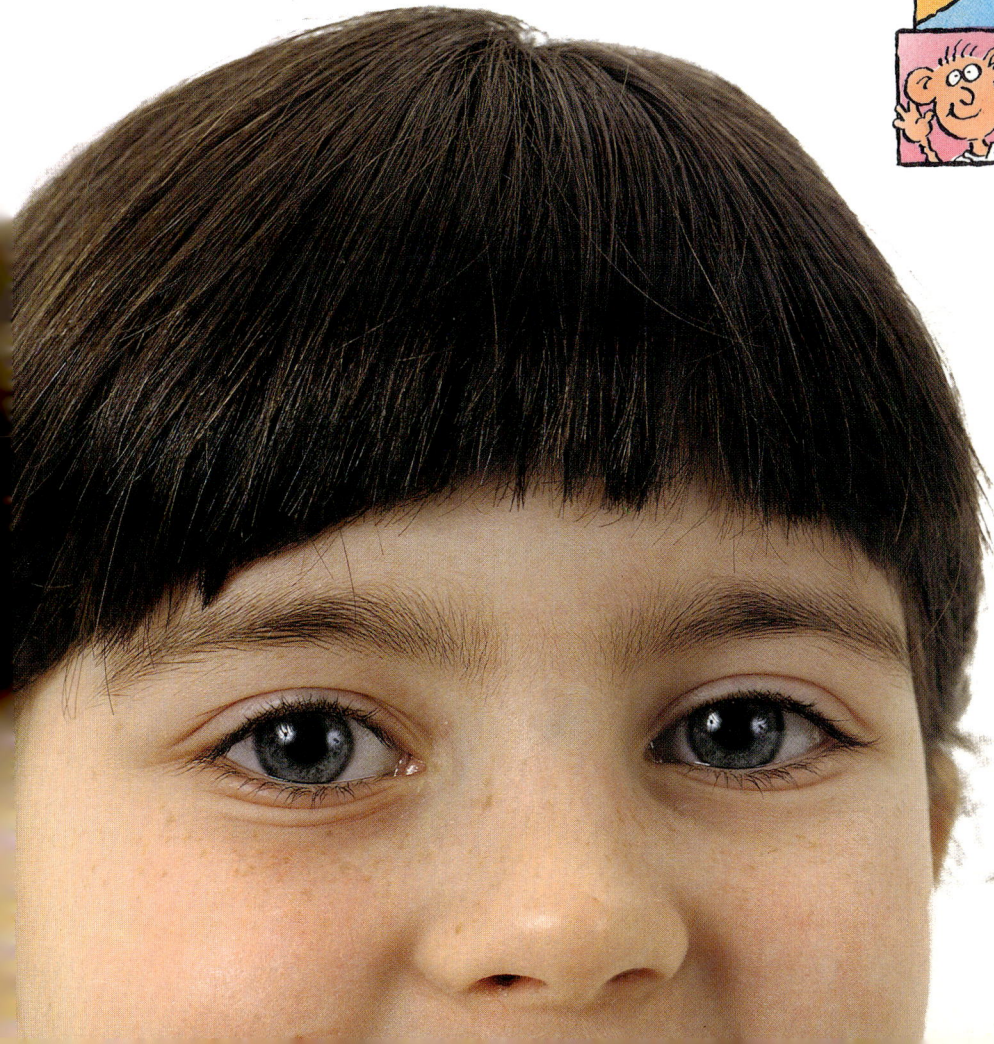

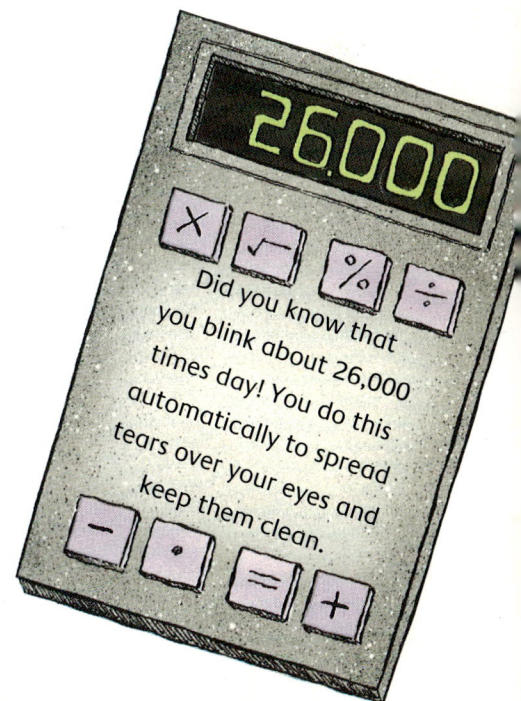

26.000

Did you know that you blink about 26,000 times day! You do this automatically to spread tears over your eyes and keep them clean.

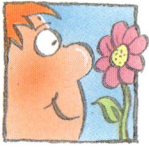

Why do I sniff to smell things properly?

Sniffing hard carries a lot of the smells in the air to the very top of your nose. This is where smells are detected and signals are sent to the brain. You can smell up to 10,000 different smells. Smells often remind you of places, or things that have happened to you.

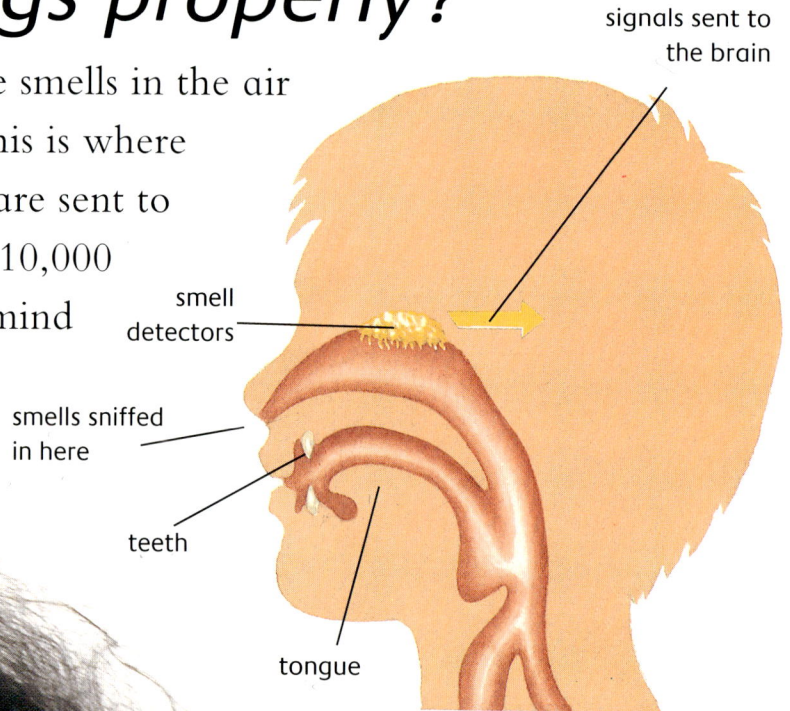

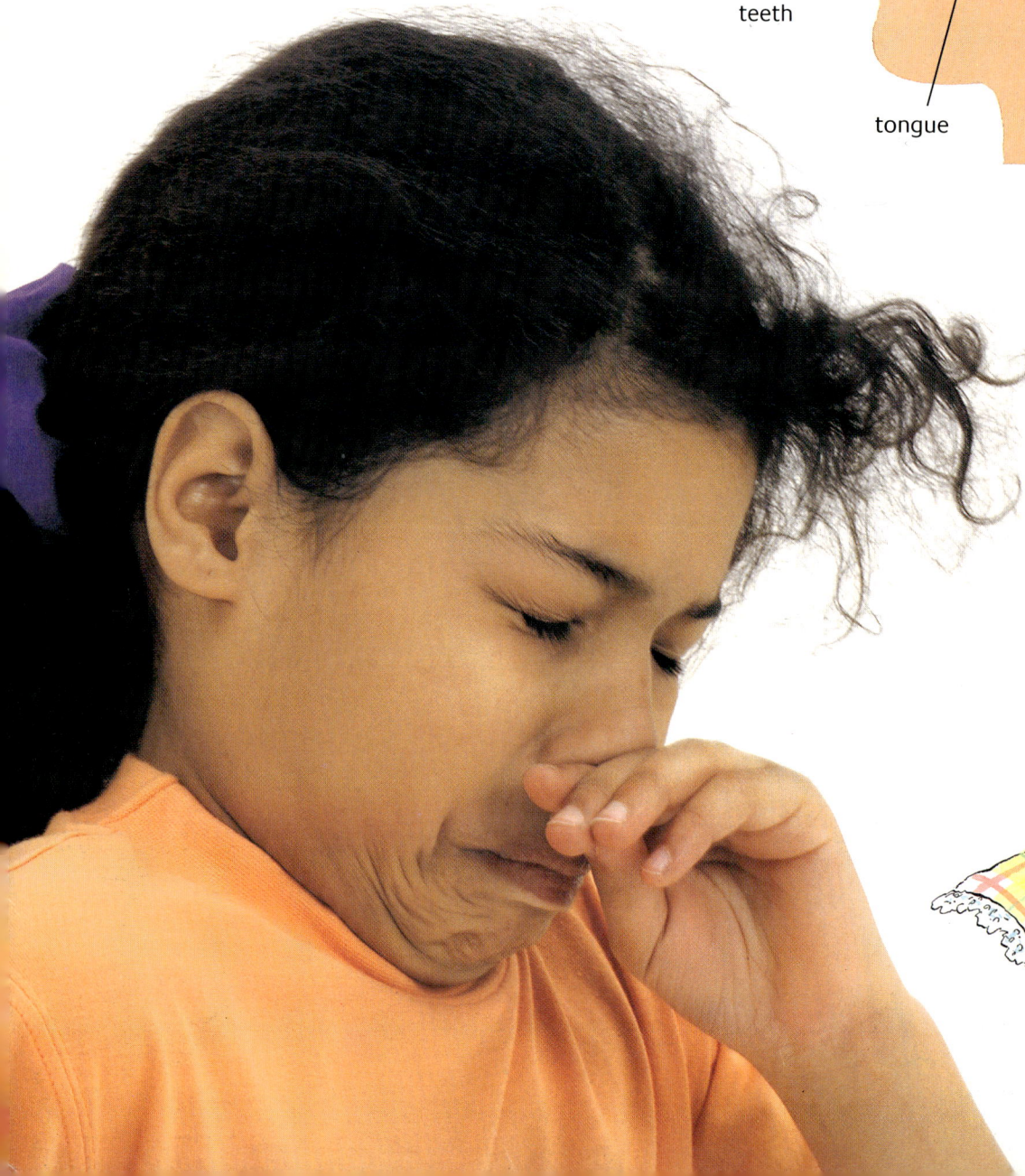

signals sent to the brain

smell detectors

smells sniffed in here

teeth

tongue

Why do I sneeze?

Sneezing gets rid of things such as dust and germs, which shouldn't be in your nose. If you have a cold, the air you sneeze out contains millions of germs. If other people breathe in your germs, they may catch your cold.

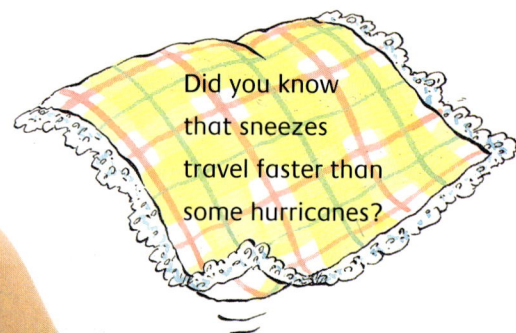

Did you know that sneezes travel faster than some hurricanes?

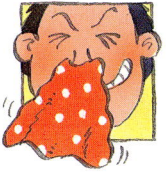

Why does my food taste funny when I've got a cold?

The taste of something depends partly on the way it smells. You can't smell properly when you have a cold, so your food tastes different. Usually it doesn't taste very nice. Your sense of smell is thousands of times more sensitive than your sense of taste.

What are the little bumps on my tongue?

Underneath the bumps on your tongue are over 10,000 taste buds. They detect the flavour of food and send messages to your brain telling you what the food tastes like.

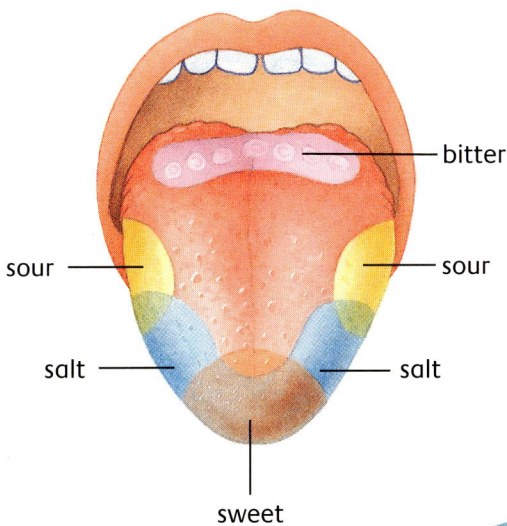

bitter

sour — sour

salt — salt

sweet

Salty and sweet tastes are detected at the front of your tongue. The taste buds for bitter tastes are at the back of your tongue.

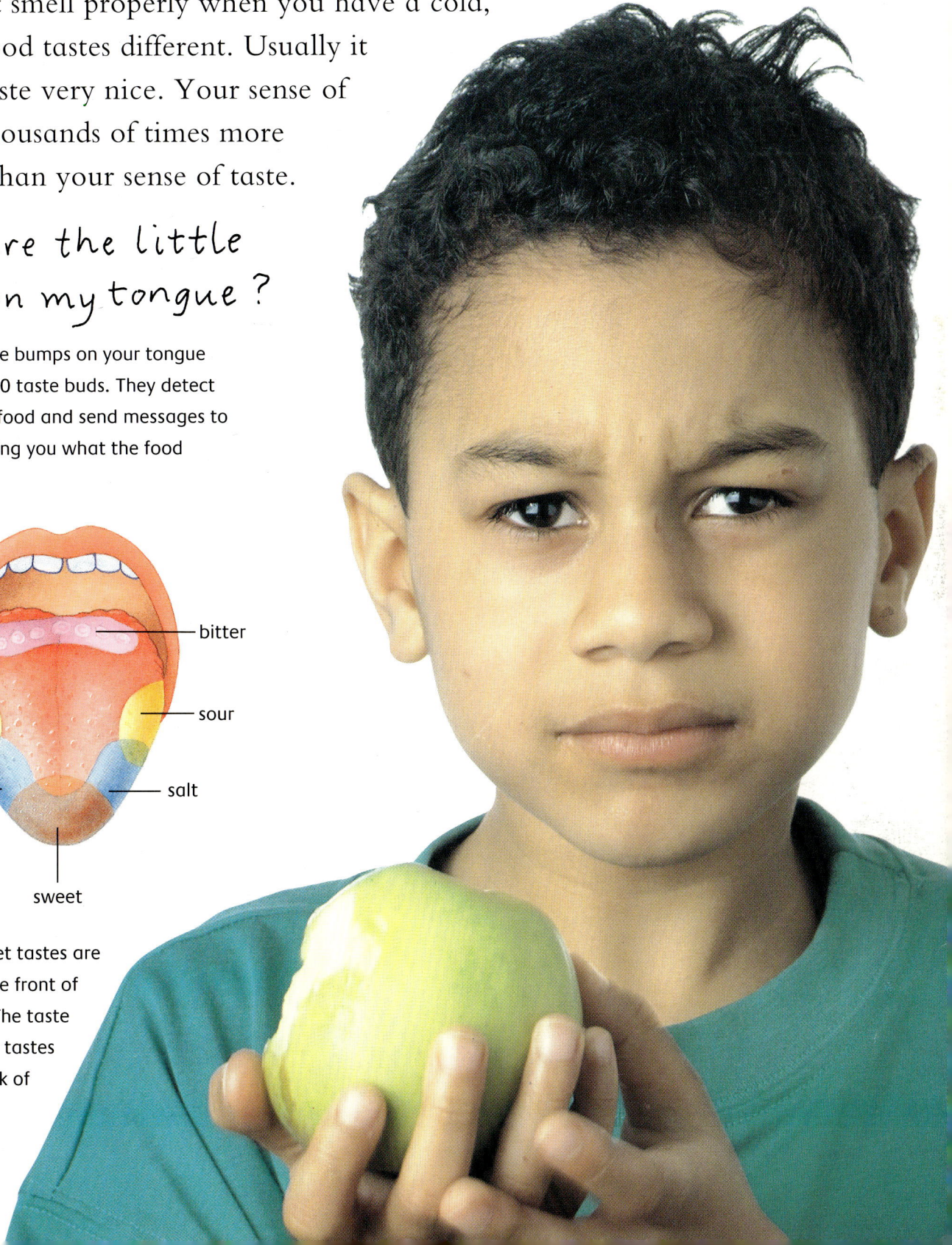

Why do my first teeth fall out?

How many first teeth do I have?

About 20. That's all there is room for in child-sized jaws. But you will have about 32 teeth eventually, when your new set of teeth comes through.

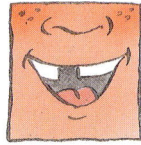

Teeth can't grow as you grow, so you have two sets of teeth. One set fits your mouth when you are a child and the other set fits your mouth when you grow bigger. Your first teeth fall out when you are between six and twelve years old. They are pushed out by the bigger teeth growing underneath them.

Why are sweets bad for my teeth?

When you eat sweets, bits of sugar get stuck in your teeth. Germs hanging around in your mouth eat up the sugar and make acid. This destroys the tough enamel coating around your teeth, making holes. If the hole goes right through to the middle of your tooth, you get toothache.

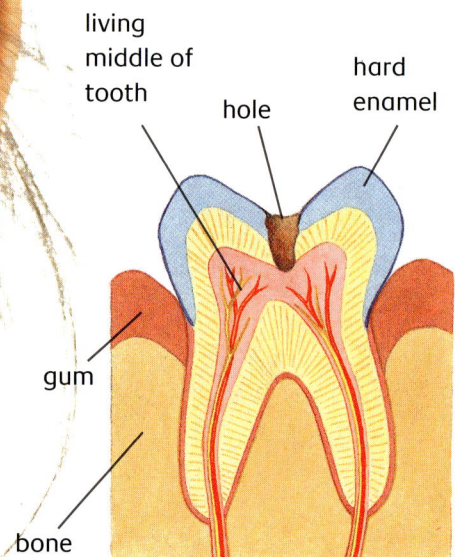

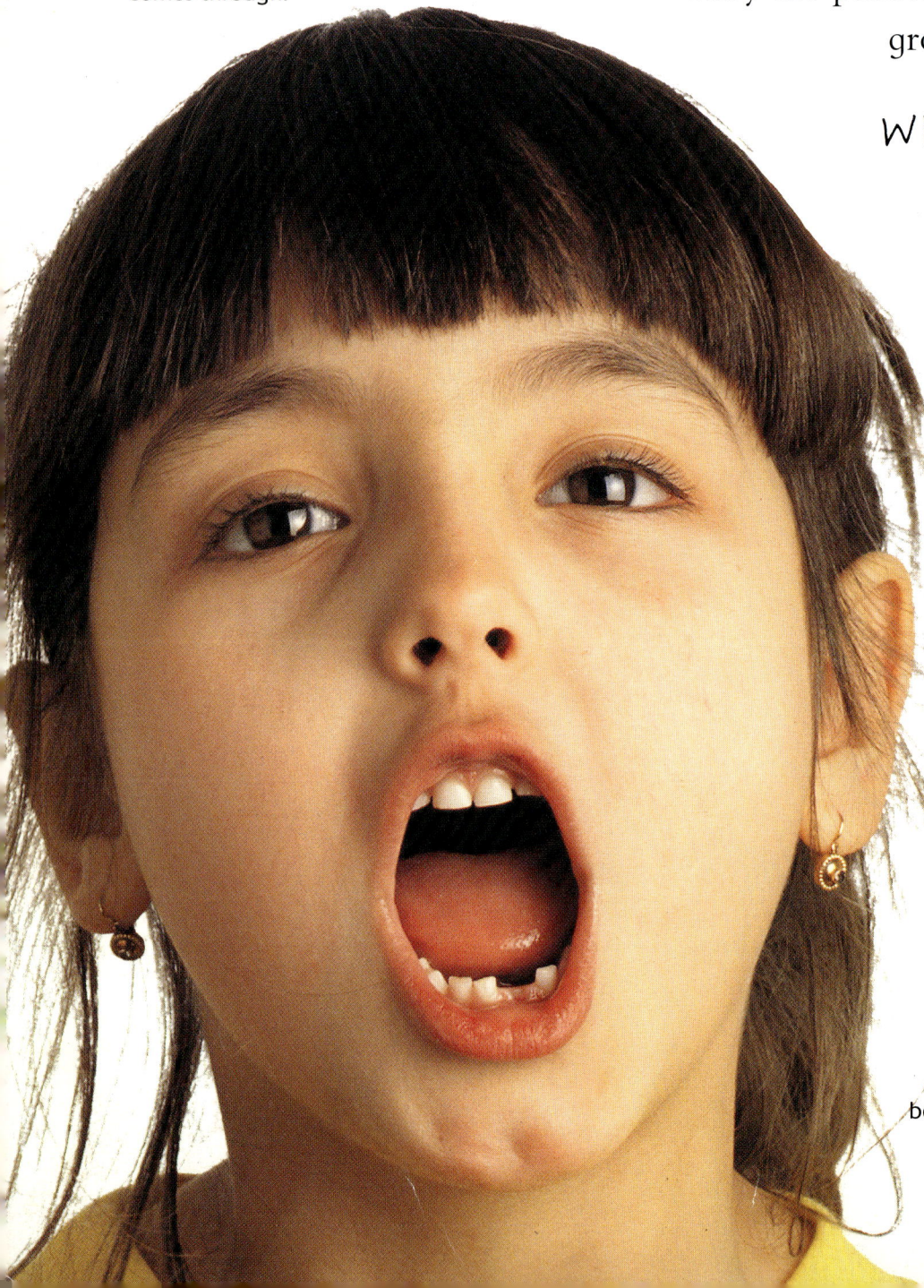

living middle of tooth

hole

hard enamel

gum

bone

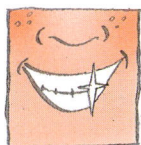

Why do I need to brush my teeth?

It's a good idea to brush your teeth at least twice a day, after breakfast and before you go to bed. Brushing gets rid of the bits of food, acid and germs and stops holes forming in your teeth. Then you won't need fillings!

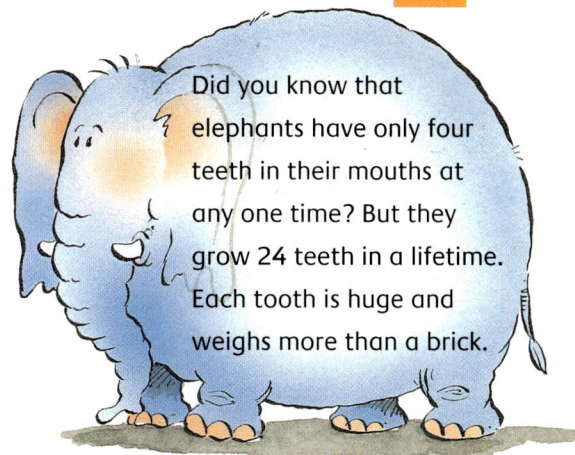

Did you know that elephants have only four teeth in their mouths at any one time? But they grow 24 teeth in a lifetime. Each tooth is huge and weighs more than a brick.

What sort of teeth do I have?

You have three main kinds of teeth to bite, chop and chew your food into pieces small enough to swallow.

sharp, scissor-like incisor teeth for biting

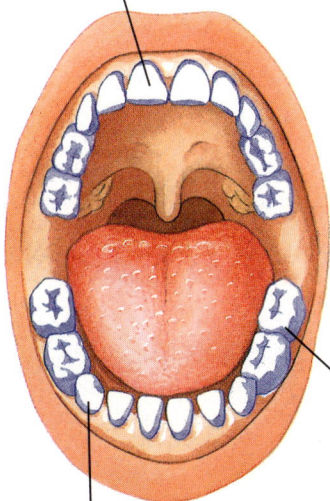

large molar teeth with ridges for grinding

pointy canine teeth for tearing and cutting

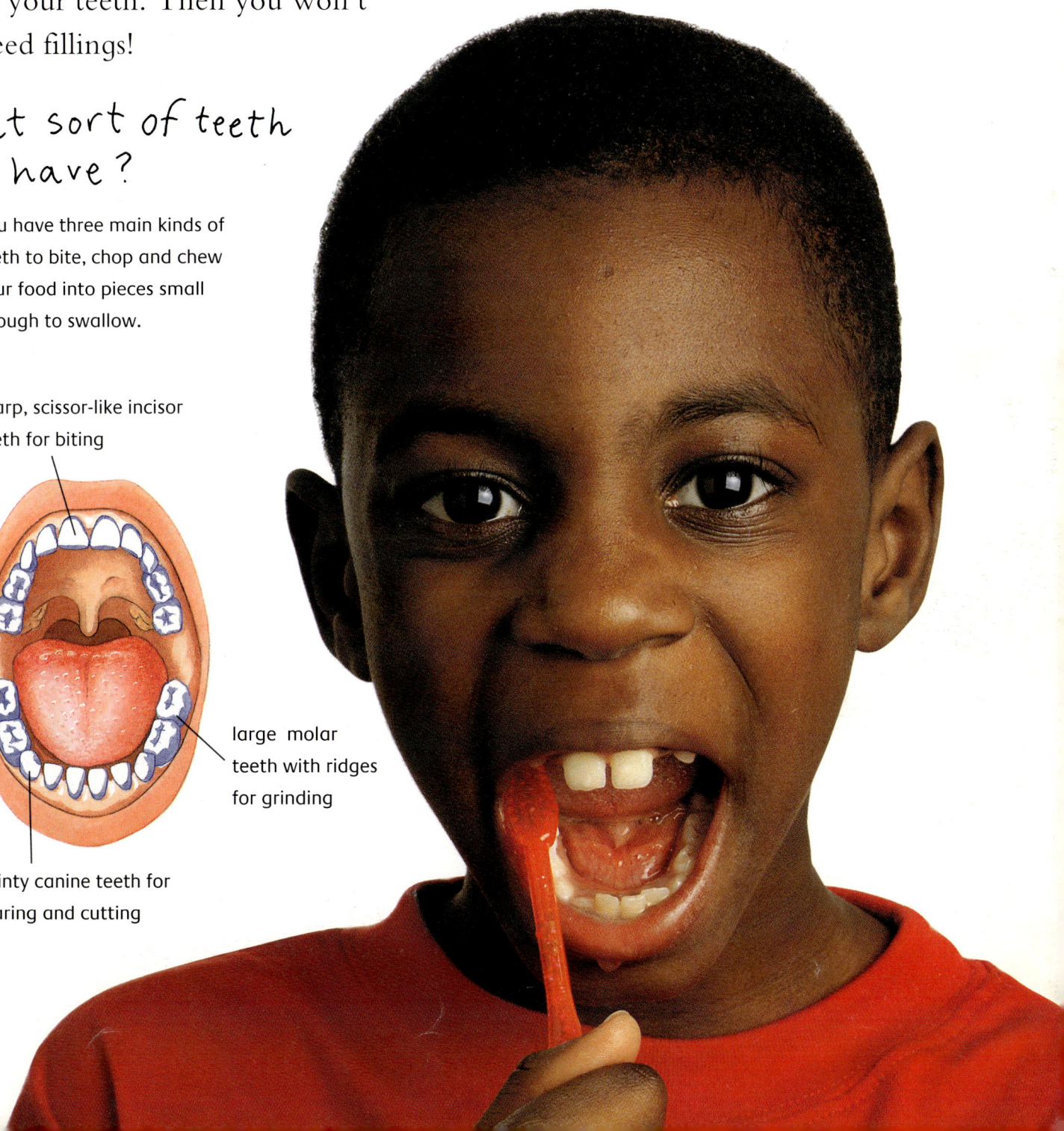

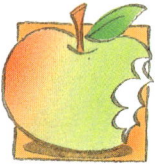

Why do I feel hungry?

Your body needs food at regular times to work properly, to grow and to keep you healthy. When your stomach is empty, it sends a signal to your brain telling you to eat something. This makes you feel hungry.

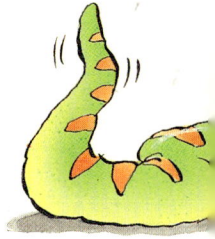

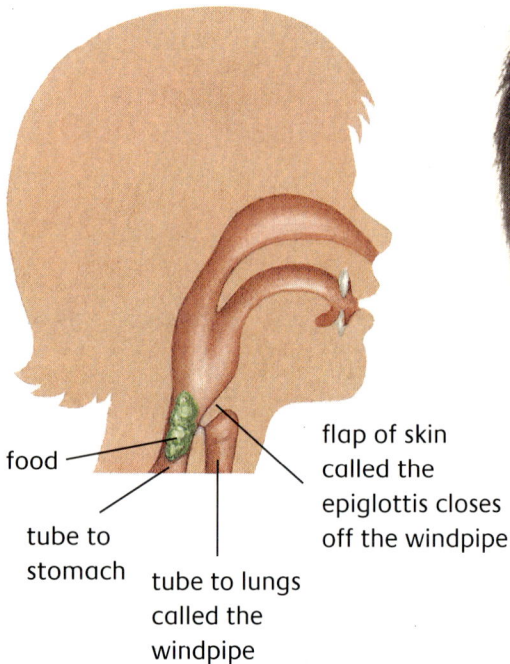

food

tube to stomach

tube to lungs called the windpipe

flap of skin called the epiglottis closes off the windpipe

Why does food go down the wrong way?

In your throat, the tube to your stomach and the tube to your lungs are very close together. When you swallow food, a flap of skin usually blocks off the tube to your lungs. But if food goes down the lung tube by mistake, it makes you choke and cough up the food. Then you can swallow it down the right way.

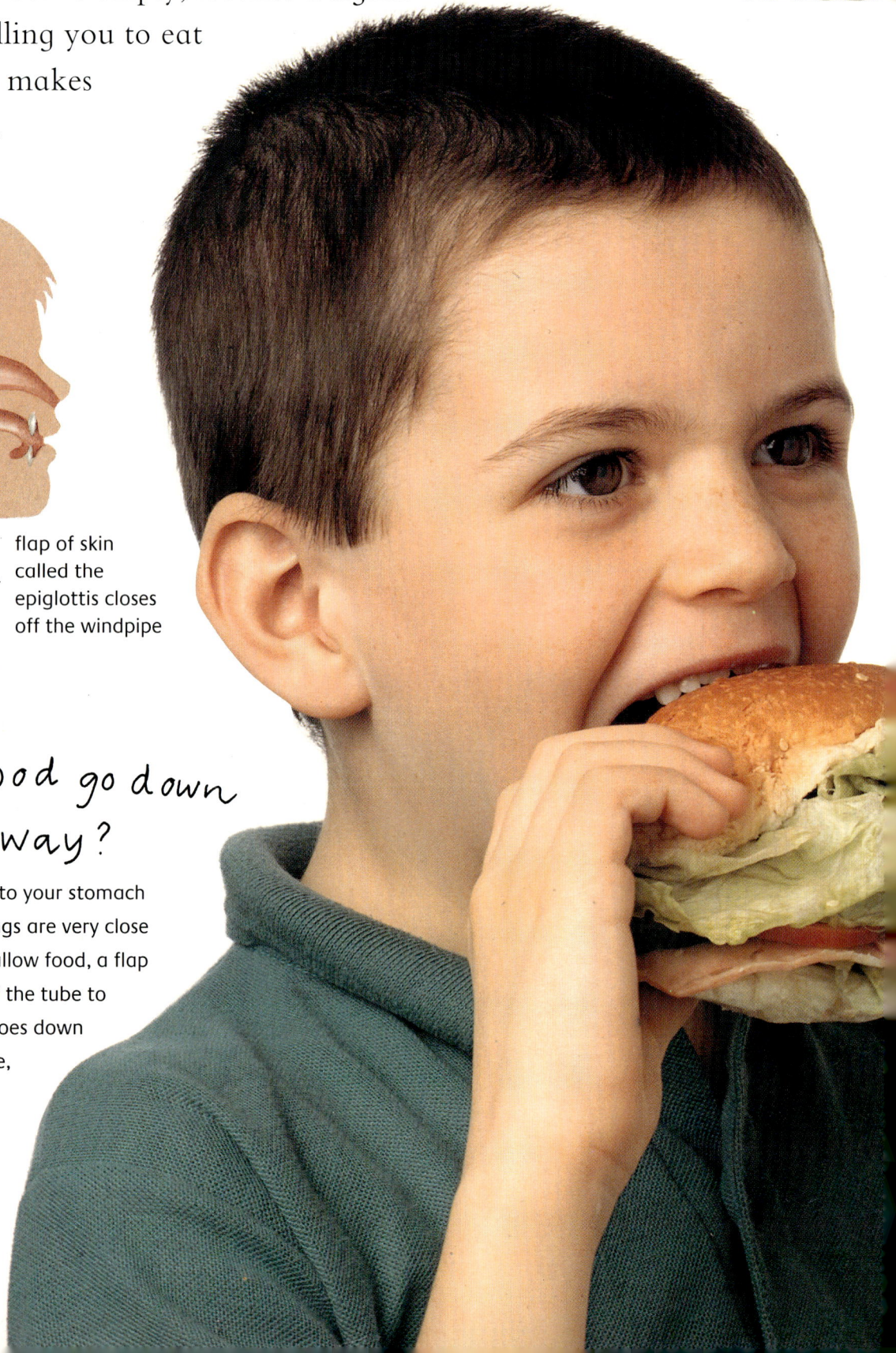

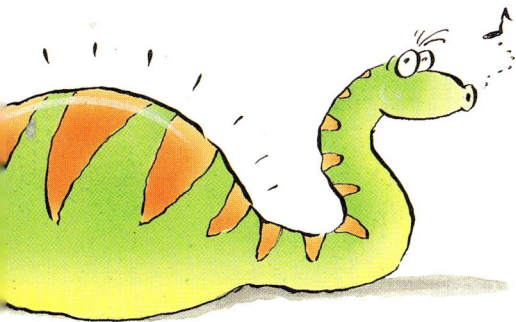

Pythons can eat a whole goat or a pig in one go. Then they don't need to eat for several months.

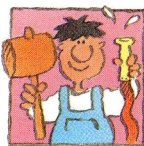

What does my stomach do?

Your stomach squeezes and squashes food and squirts juices over it until it turns into a mushy soup. Food has to be broken down into smaller pieces so it can be taken into your blood and carried around your body to where it is needed.

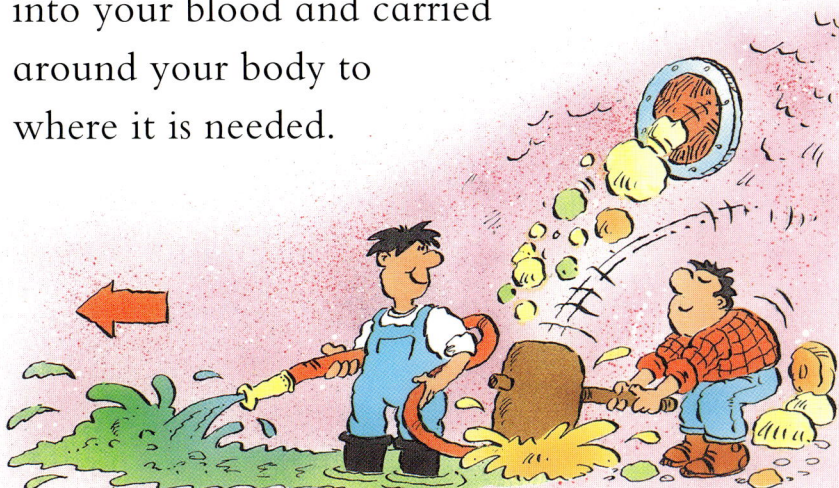

How big is my stomach?

Your stomach can hold up to 15 cupfuls of food at any one time. It is a stretchy bag shaped like the letter 'J'.

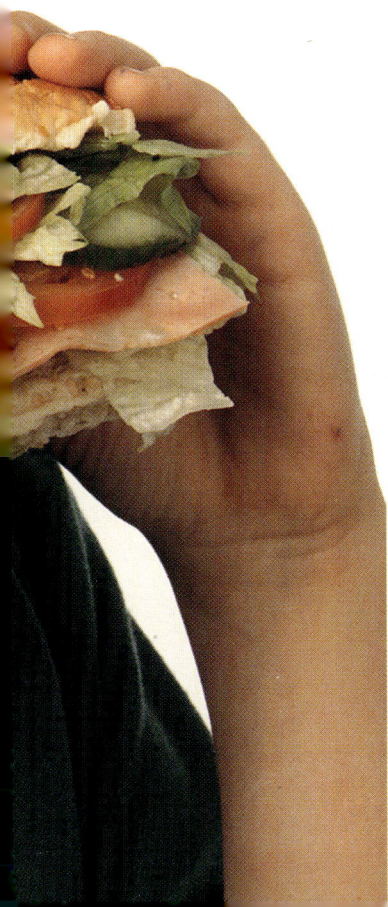

True or false?

1 Eating an apple gives you enough energy to swim for 2 hours.

2 Food stays in the stomach for 2 – 6 hours.

3 A person eats about 50 tonnes of food in a lifetime. That weighs as much as 6 elephants!

4 A cow has 5 stomachs.

5 Green potatoes are poisonous.

The answers are on page 32.

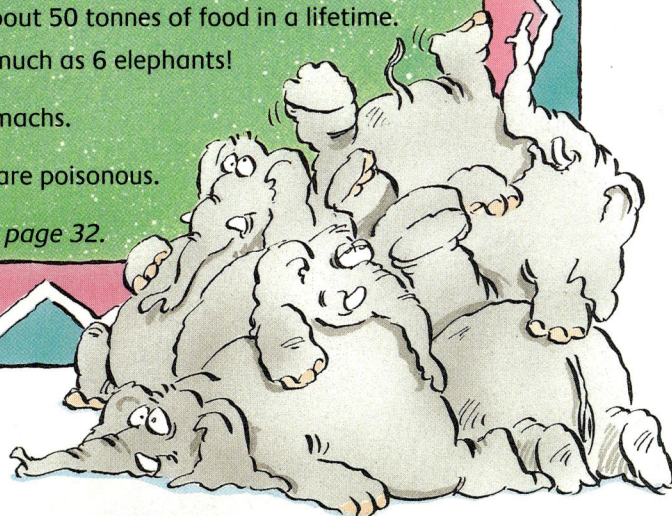

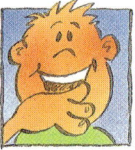

Why do I burp?

Sometimes, when you swallow food too quickly or drink fizzy drinks, you swallow a lot of air as well. Then when the stomach stirs up the food or drink, the air gets pushed back into your mouth. It comes out as a burp.

What makes my mouth water?

When you chew food, or even think about eating, saliva or spit floods into your mouth. Saliva makes food soft and moist, so it is easy to swallow.

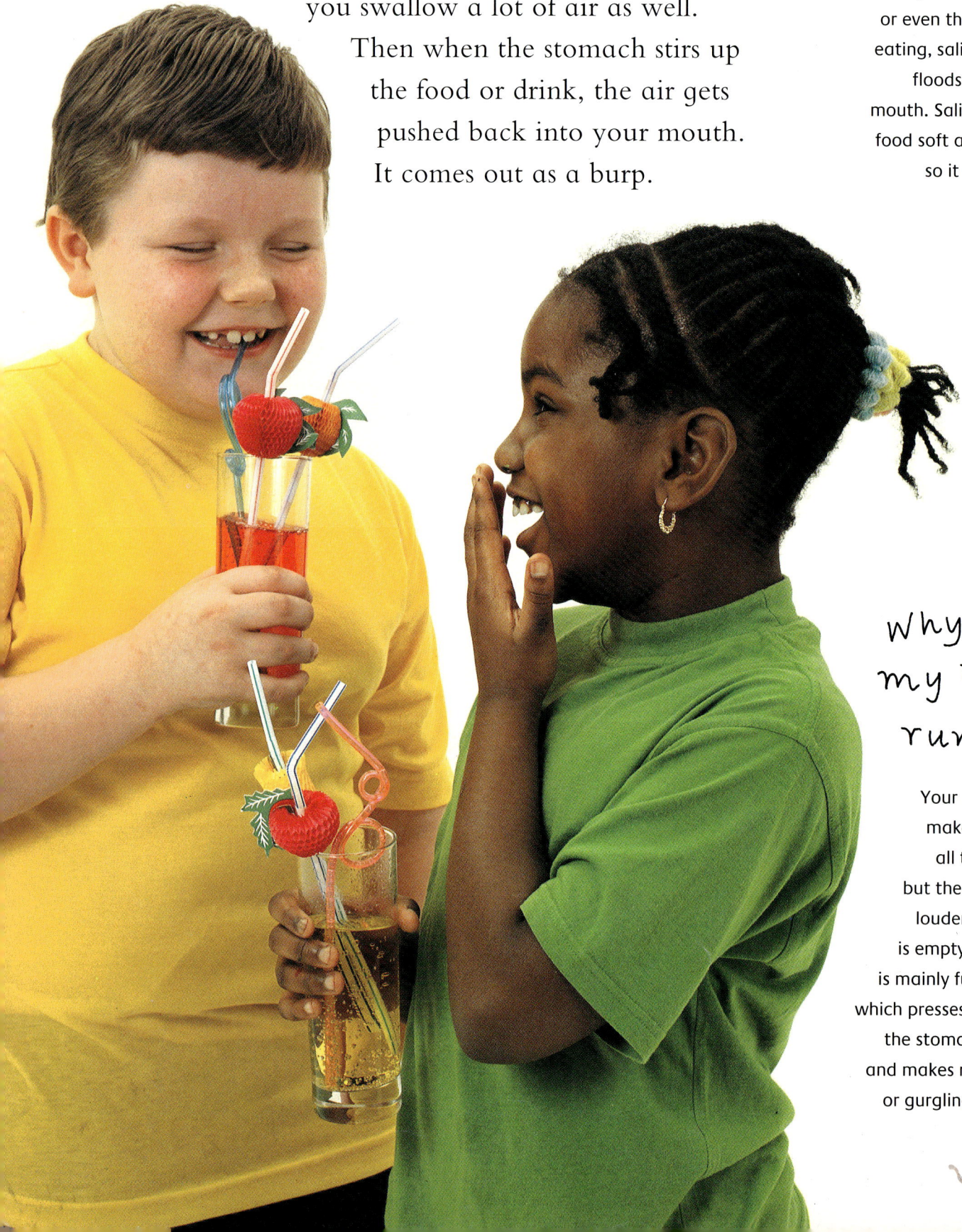

Why does my tummy rumble?

Your stomach makes noises all the time, but these sound louder when it is empty. Then it is mainly full of air, which presses against the stomach walls and makes rumbling or gurgling noises.

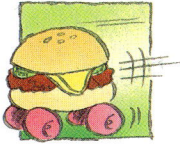

How does food move through my body?

Muscles push food through tubes inside your body. These muscles can push food up as well as down, so you could eat standing on your head. (But don't try it, you might choke.)

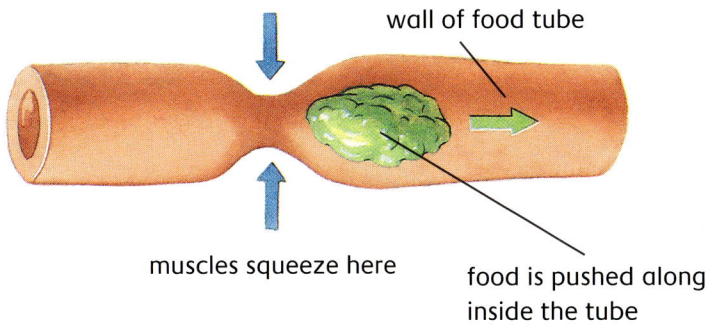

wall of food tube

muscles squeeze here

food is pushed along inside the tube

what happens to food inside me?

Did you know that if all the food pipes inside your body were stretched out, they would be as long as three cars?

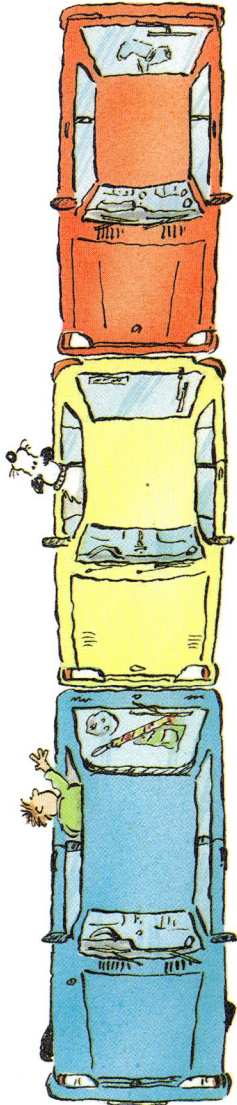

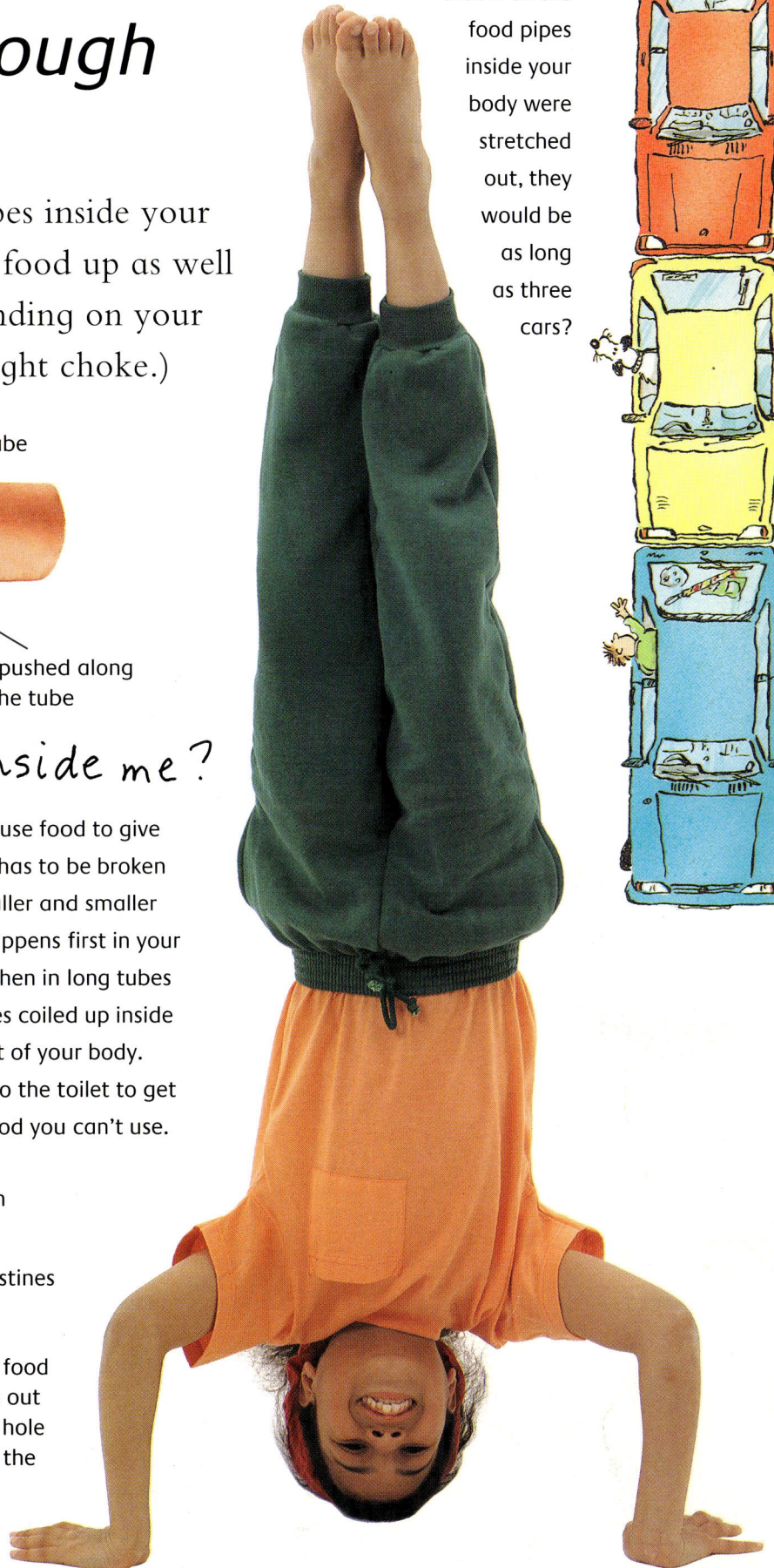

Before you can use food to give you energy, it has to be broken down into smaller and smaller pieces. This happens first in your stomach and then in long tubes called intestines coiled up inside the middle bit of your body.

You go to the toilet to get rid of food you can't use.

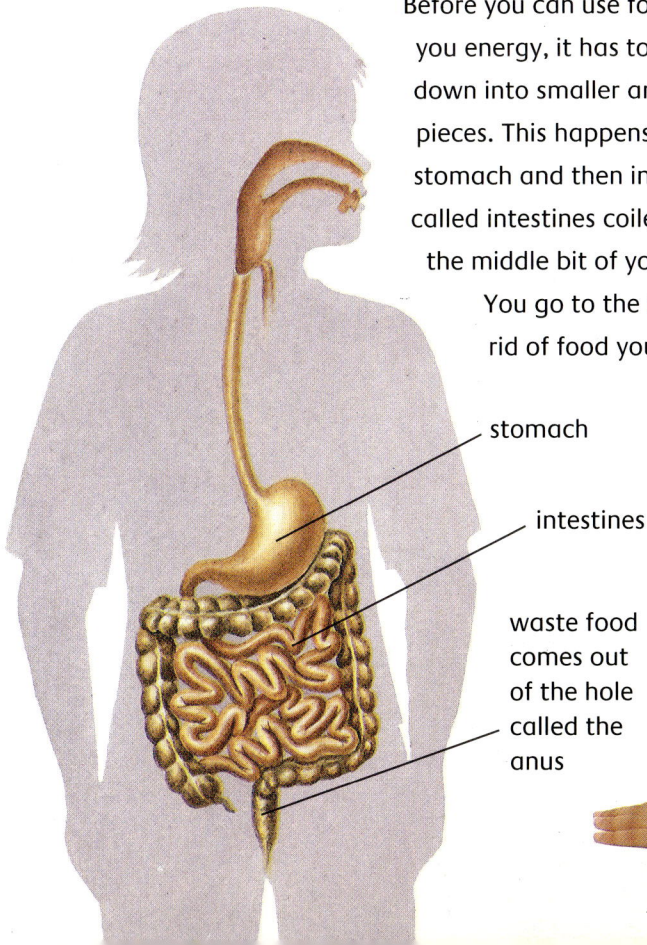

stomach

intestines

waste food comes out of the hole called the anus

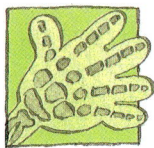

What do bones do?

Bones help you to stand up and move about. They give your body its shape – like the poles in a tent – and protect your insides from injury. Without bones, you would be as squidgy as a jelly. Bones can't move on their own, but muscles are joined onto bones and pull them to and fro.

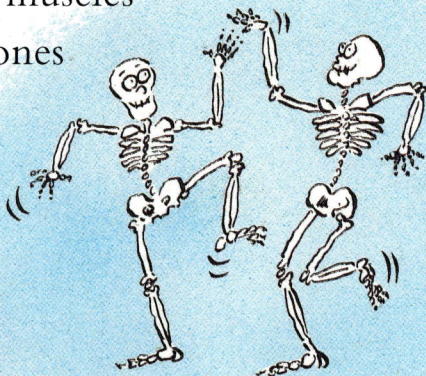

Did you know that your biggest muscles are in your thighs and in your bottom? You have about 649 muscles in your body.

About half of all your bones are in your feet and your hands – 26 in each foot and 27 in each hand.

2 toe bones called phalanges in your big toe

5 sole bones called metatarsals

3 phalanges in each other toe

7 ankle bones called tarsals

How many bones do I have?

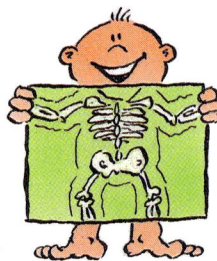

You have 206 bones, but when you were a baby, you had over 300 bones. Some of a baby's bones join together as it grows up.

What is my funny bone?

Your funny bone is not a bone at all really. Just a place on your elbow where you feel pain easily. So if you bang your elbow at this spot, a sharp pain shoots up your arm.

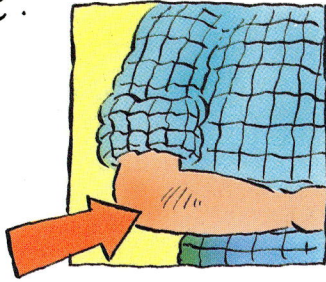

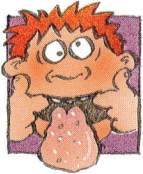

What is cramp?

If you go swimming or running after a meal, you may get cramp. This could be because a lot of energy is being used to break down your meal. There is not enough energy left to power your muscles.

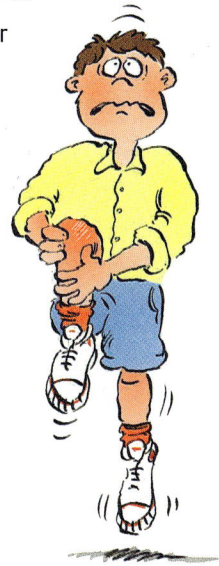

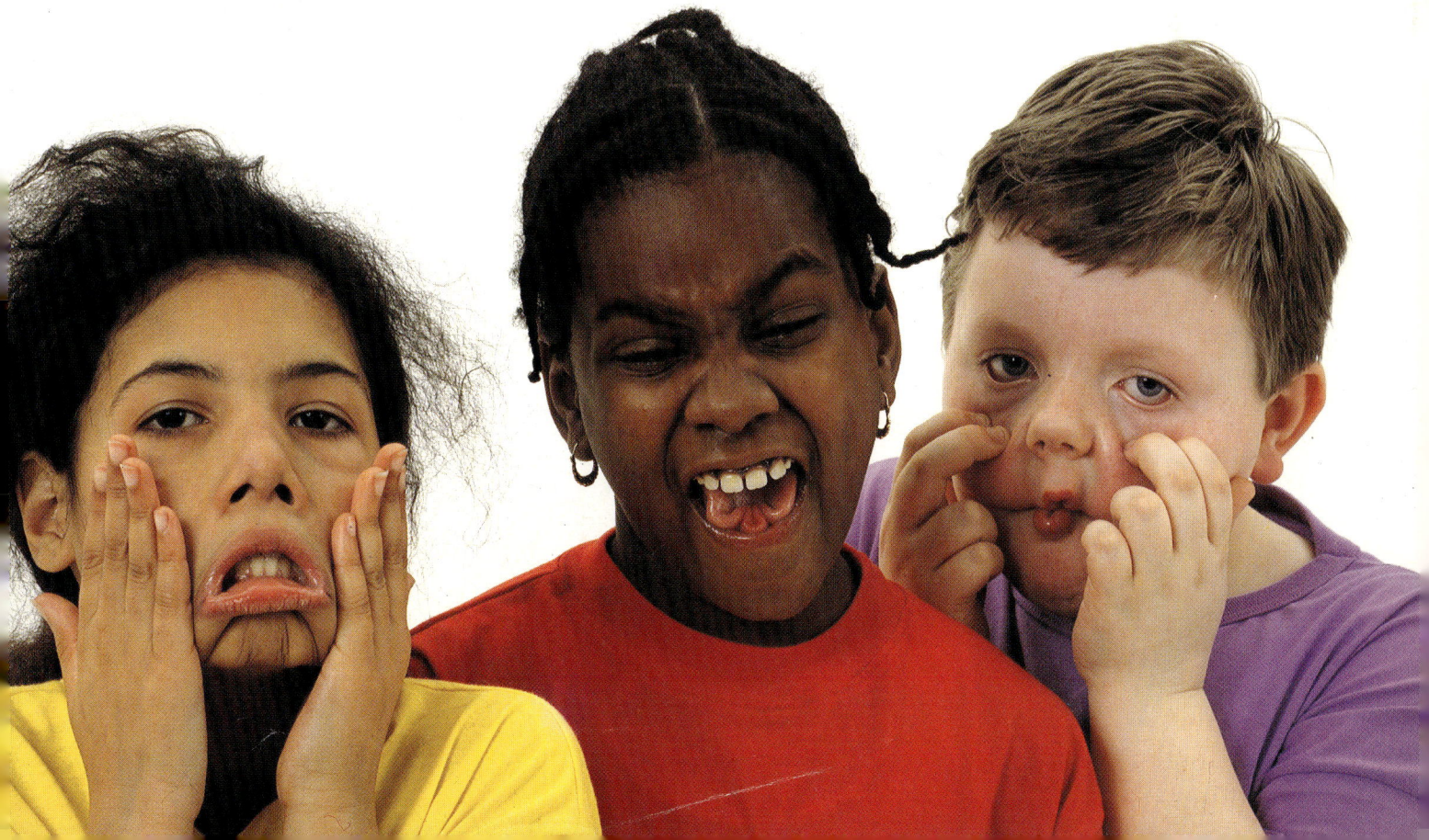

What happens when I pull faces?

You have about 30 muscles under the skin on your face. They pull the skin to make you smile, frown or raise your eyebrows. When you smile, you use about 15 different muscles. Even when you are not pulling faces, the muscles work to hold your face in place.

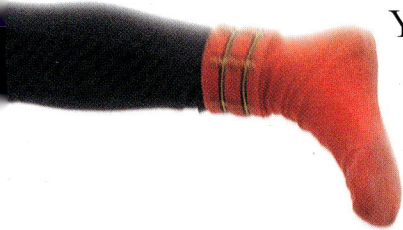

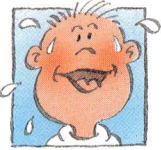

Why do I pant if I run fast?

You need a lot of energy if you run fast. And the air you breathe sets free energy from your food. So if you pant, you take in more air to give you more energy. When you stop running, you may go on breathing extra fast for a little while to make up for all the air you used up in running.

Breathing in

air in

tube to lungs

lungs

diaphragm down

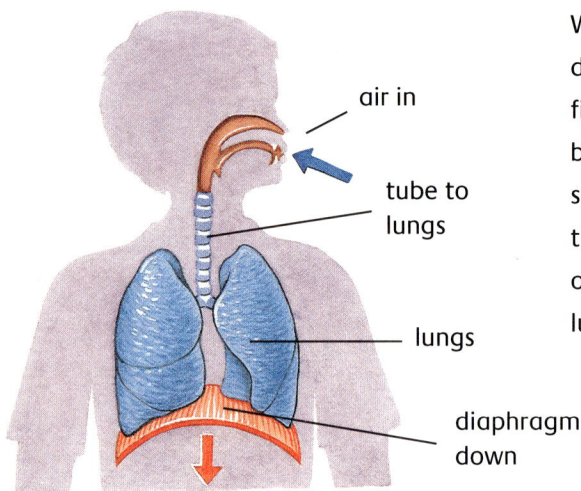

How do I breathe?

When you breathe in, the diaphragm moves down and air fills your lungs. When you breathe out, the diaphragm springs back up and this pushes the air out of your lungs again.

Breathing out

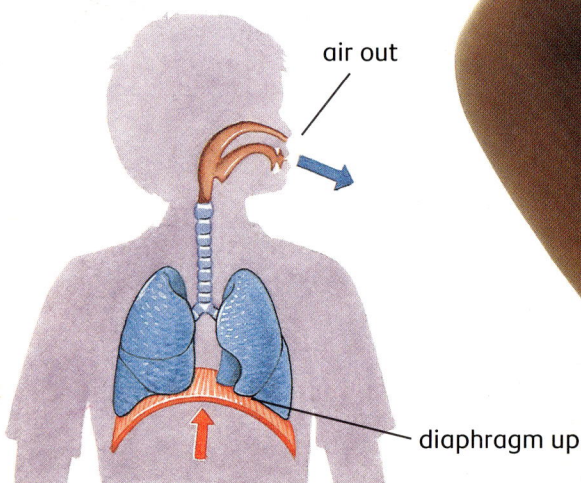

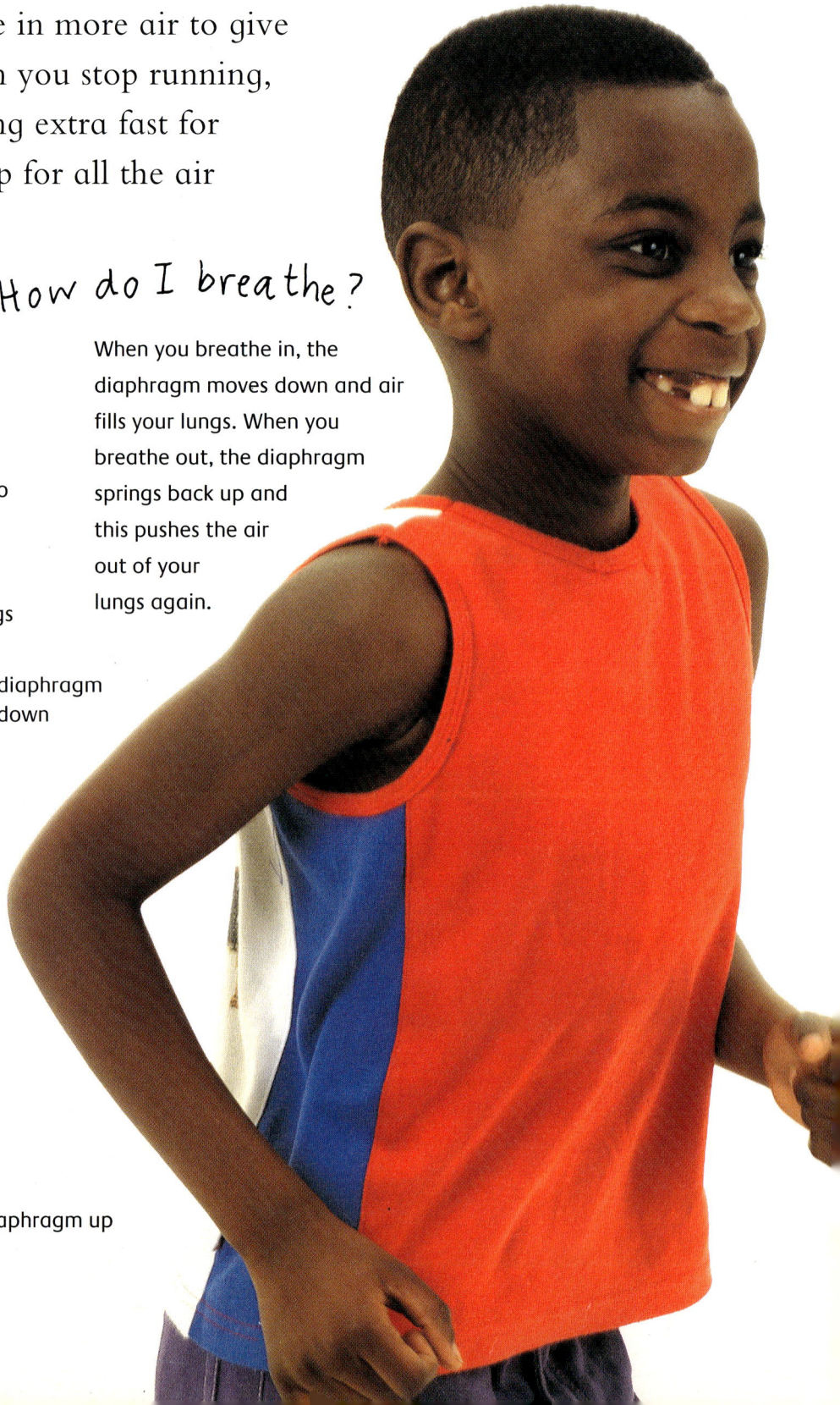

air out

diaphragm up

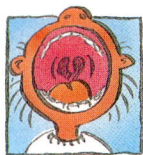

Where does my voice come from?

It comes from the knobbly lump in your throat called the Adam's apple. Stretched across this lump are two flaps called vocal cords. When you breathe out, the air going through the cords makes them wobble – it's rather like twanging an elastic band. Your lips, tongue, cheeks and throat shape the sounds into words.

Why do I yawn?

No-one is quite sure. It may be a way of getting more fresh air to the brain if you are feeling sleepy or bored. Once a yawn starts, you can't stop it even if you shut your mouth. You may yawn if you see someone else yawning – it seems to be catching!

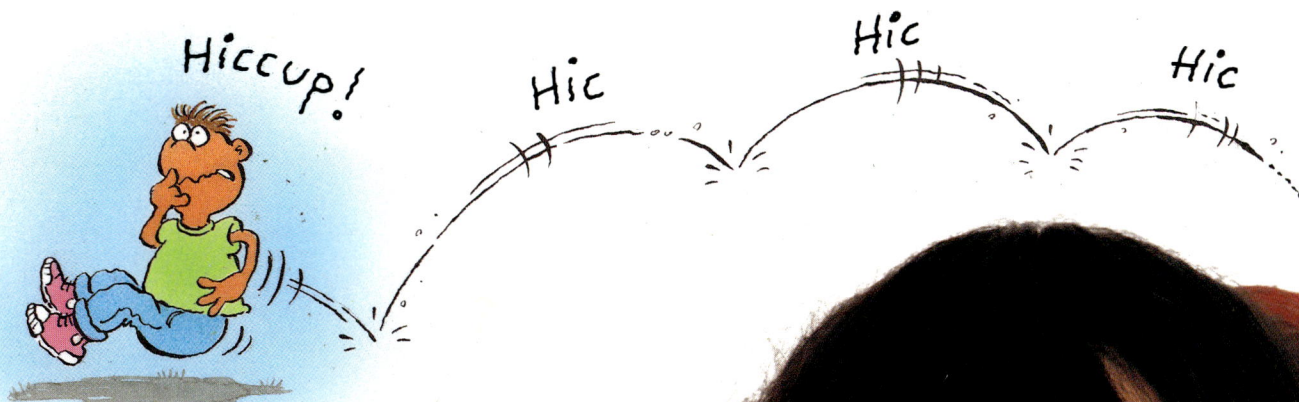

Hiccup!

Hic

Hic

Hic

Why do I get hiccups?

Hiccups happen when your diaphragm suddenly pulls down really hard, drawing lots of air into your lungs. No-one is sure why this happens. The 'hic' sound somes from air rushing in and the 'cup' sound is the flap across the tube to the lungs flapping shut suddenly. Babies may get hiccups before they are born.

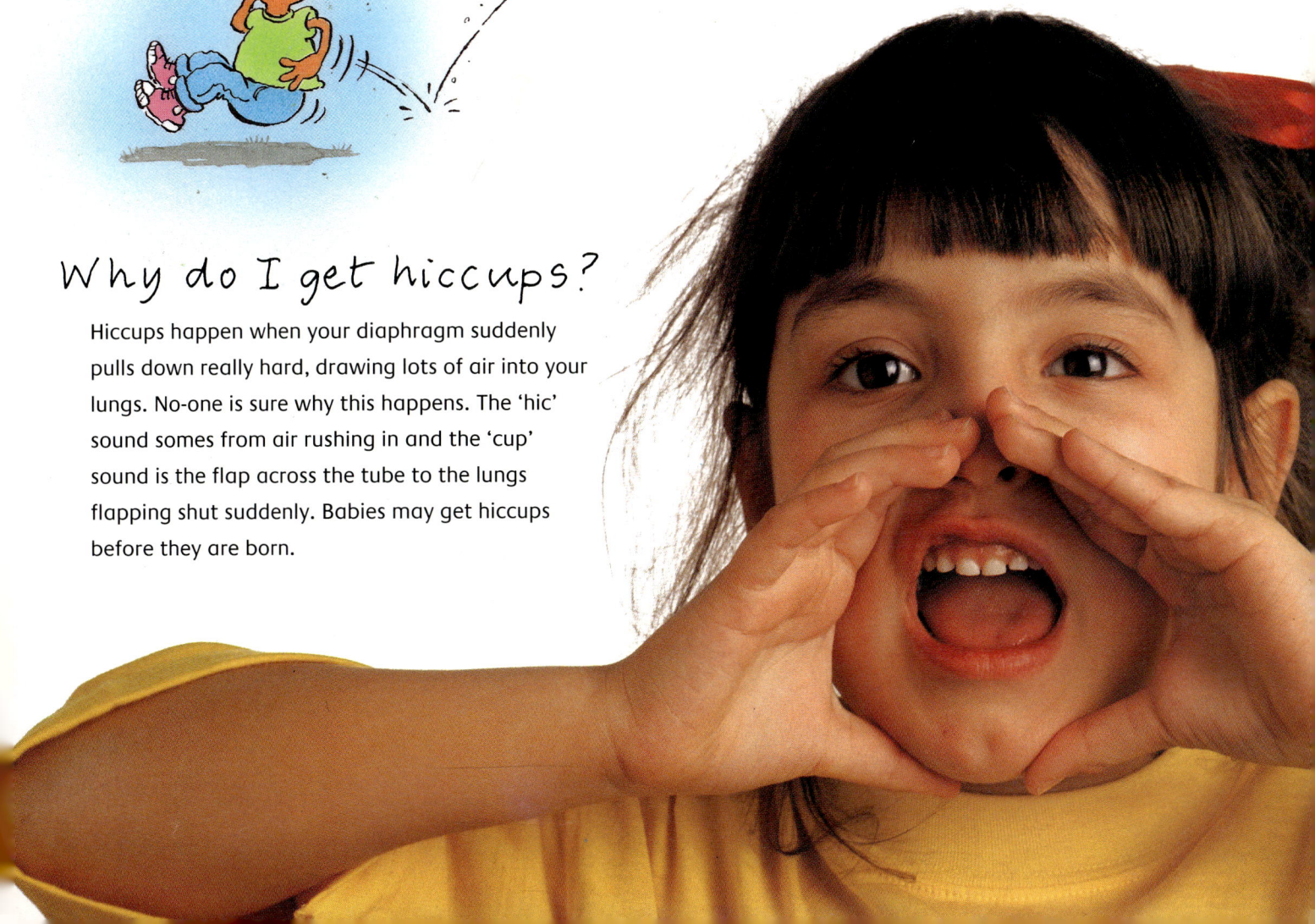

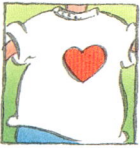

What are heartbeats?

The sound of someone's heart beating is made by little gates in the heart called valves. These slam shut after blood is pumped through them, making a thump, thump sound. This is what doctors listen to when they hold a stethoscope against your chest. They can tell from the sound if the heart is working properly.

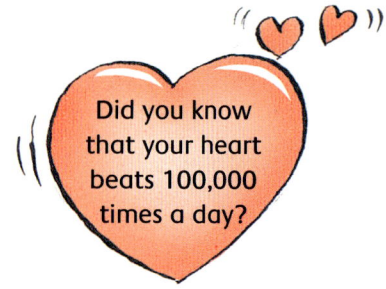

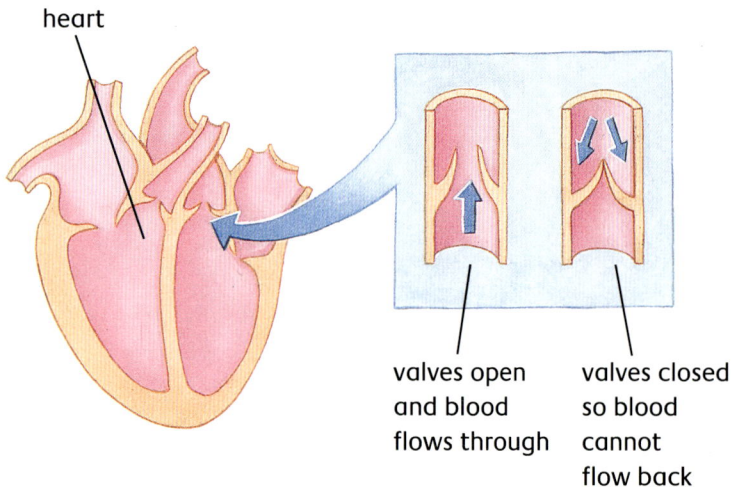

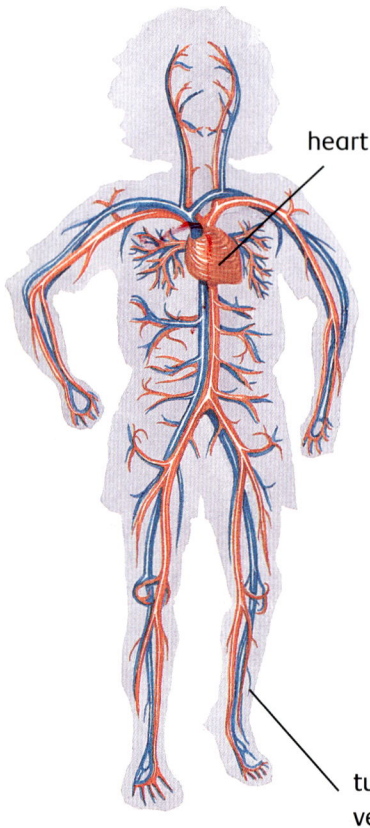

Did you know that your heart beats 100,000 times a day?

heart

valves open and blood flows through

valves closed so blood cannot flow back

heart

What does blood do?

Blood has lots of different jobs. It carries food, water and oxygen around the body. It collects unwanted food, water and other wastes so they can be pushed out of the body. And it fights germs and keeps the body at a steady temperature.

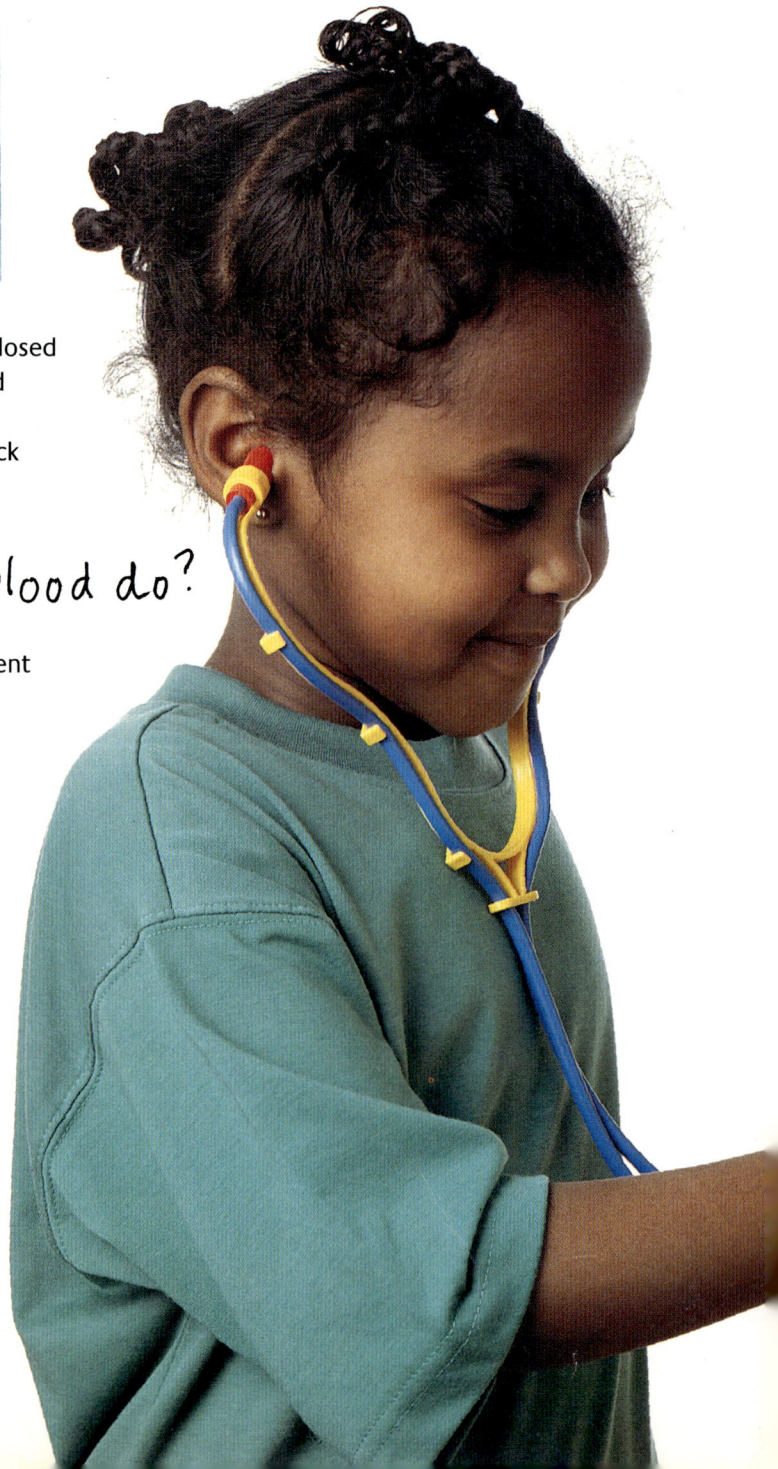

tubes called blood vessels all over the body

True or false?

1 A mouse's heart beats 10 times a minute.

2 An adult's heart weighs as much as a large potato.

3 If all the tubes that carry your blood were joined end to end, they would stretch two and a half times around the world.

4 A baby's heart starts to beat when it is inside its mother at about one month old.

The answers are on page 32.

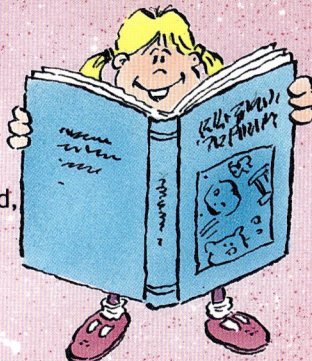

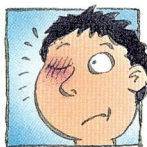

What is a bruise?

When you knock into something, some of the blood vessels under the skin may break open. Blood leaks out, making the skin look bluish-red. Eventually, the blood vessels seal up again and the skin goes back to its normal colour.

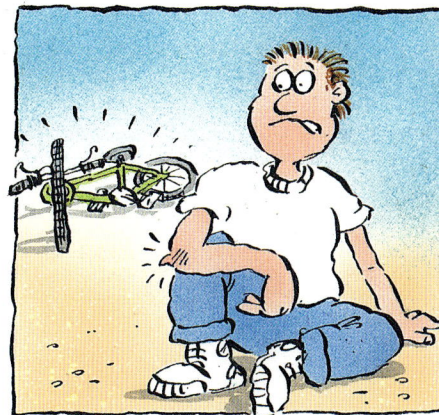

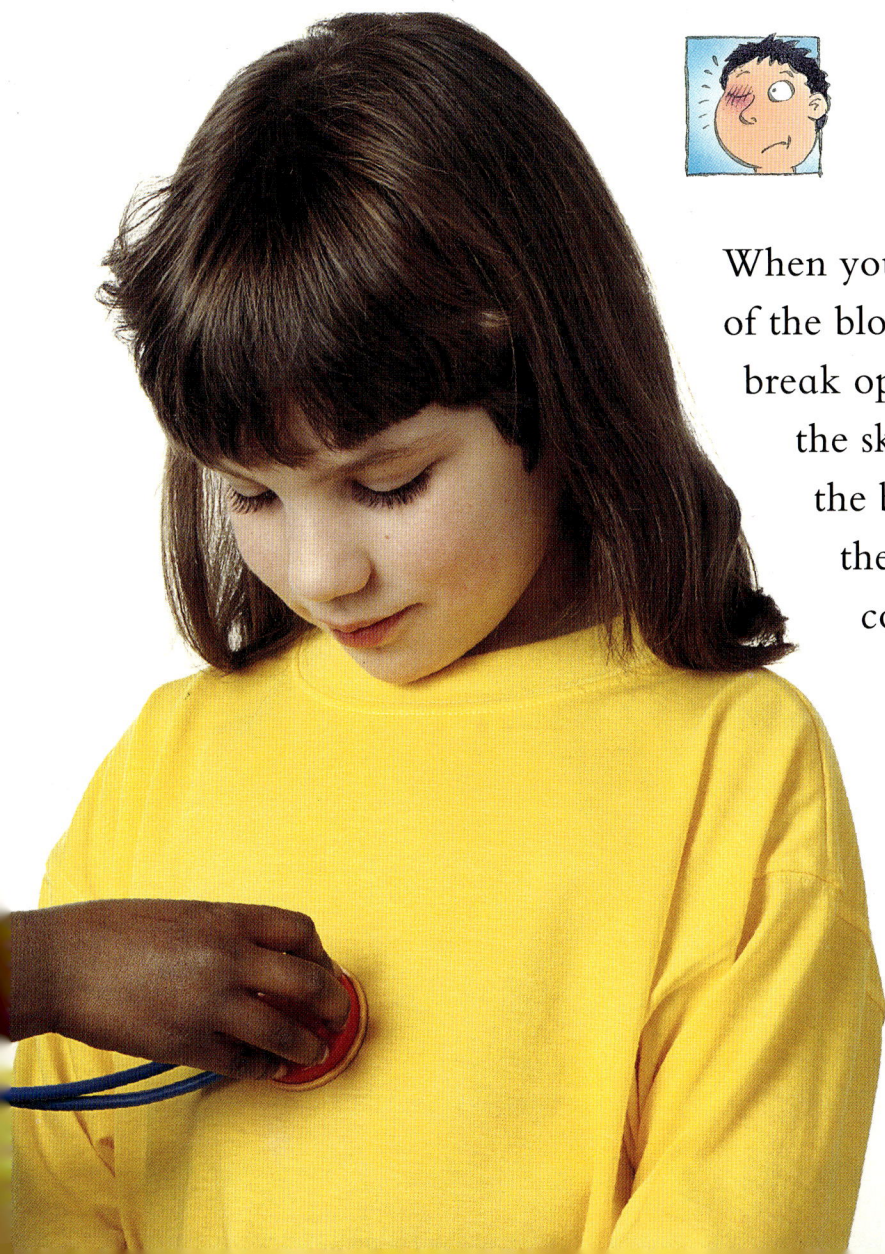

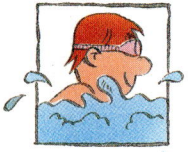

How can I keep healthy?

To keep fit and healthy you need to eat the right sorts of food, get enough rest and sleep, and take plenty of exercise. A healthy body can fight off most germs and diseases, but sometimes people need medicines to make them well again.

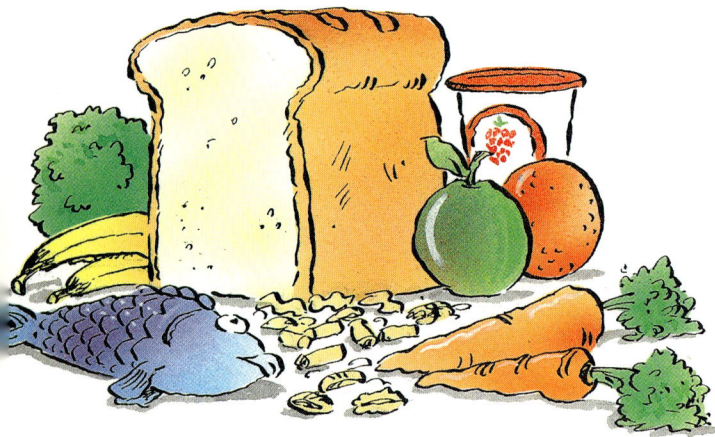

Do you know why you often feel hot when you are ill? It's because your body heats itself up to kill off the germs that are making you ill.

Why do babies need injections?

The injections contain dead or weak germs. As the babies fight off the germs, they build up a resistance to them. If they come across the strong germs when they are older, they should be able to fight them off without being really ill.

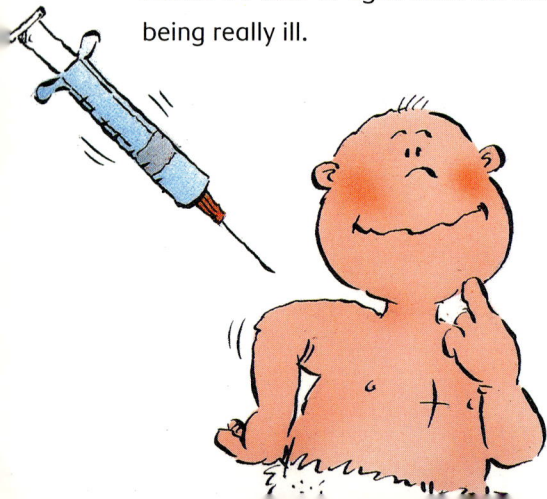

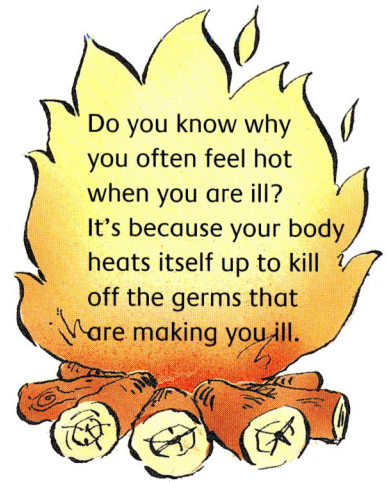

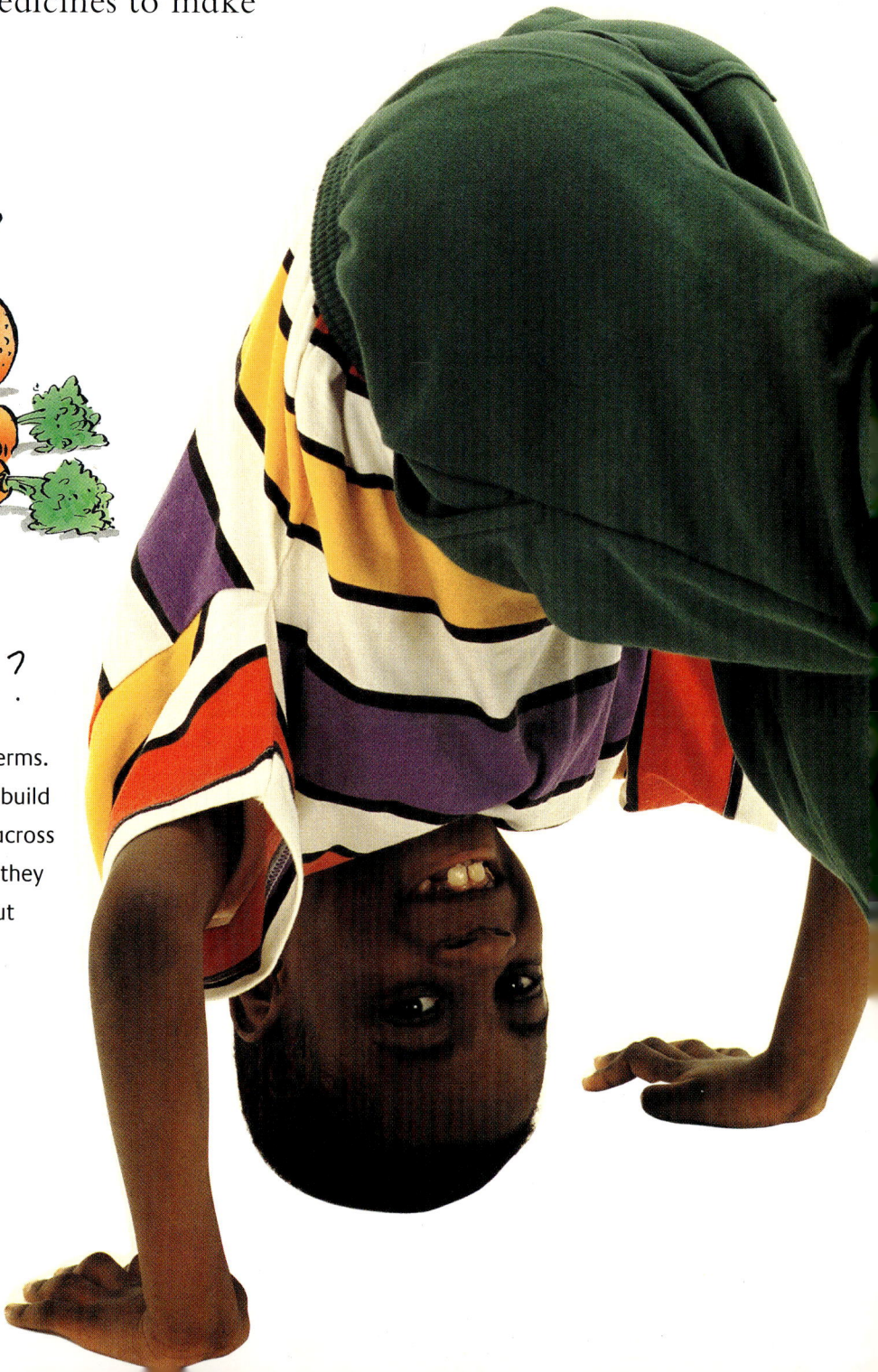

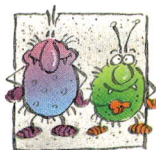

Why do I get an upset tummy?

Sometimes germs get into the stomach and the stomach doesn't want to do its job any more. The germs may come from food that has gone bad or from dirt on your hands. The stomach pushes food back the way it came, making you sick. Once you have got rid of the germs, you feel better.

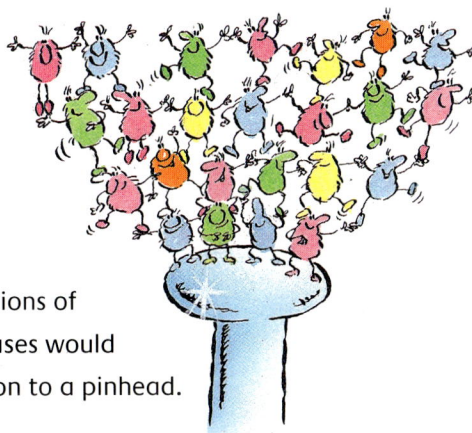

Millions of viruses would fit on to a pinhead.

What are germs?

Tiny living things, such as bacteria or viruses, which are all around you – in the air, on your skin and on the food you eat. Most germs can't hurt you but some cause illnesses such as colds, flu and tummy upsets. Germs get into your body through your nose or mouth or cuts in your skin.

True or false?

1 Fatty foods such as biscuits, fried food and chocolate are good for you.

2 When you exercise, your heart beats at up to 200 times a minute.

3 The best all-round exercise is swimming.

4 Children need less sleep than adults.

The answers are on page 32.

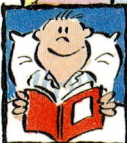

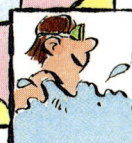

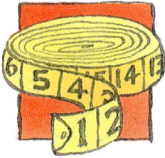

How big will I grow?

Chemical codes called genes inside your body control how big you will grow. Everyone grows at their own pace and some people grow taller than others. But good food, rest and exercise will help you grow to the maximum possible height fixed by your genes. A lot of fast growing goes on while you are asleep.

When will I stop growing?

Your body goes on growing until you are about 20 years old.

A girl who is seven and a half years old is about three quarters of the height she will be as an adult. A boy reaches this point at about nine years old.

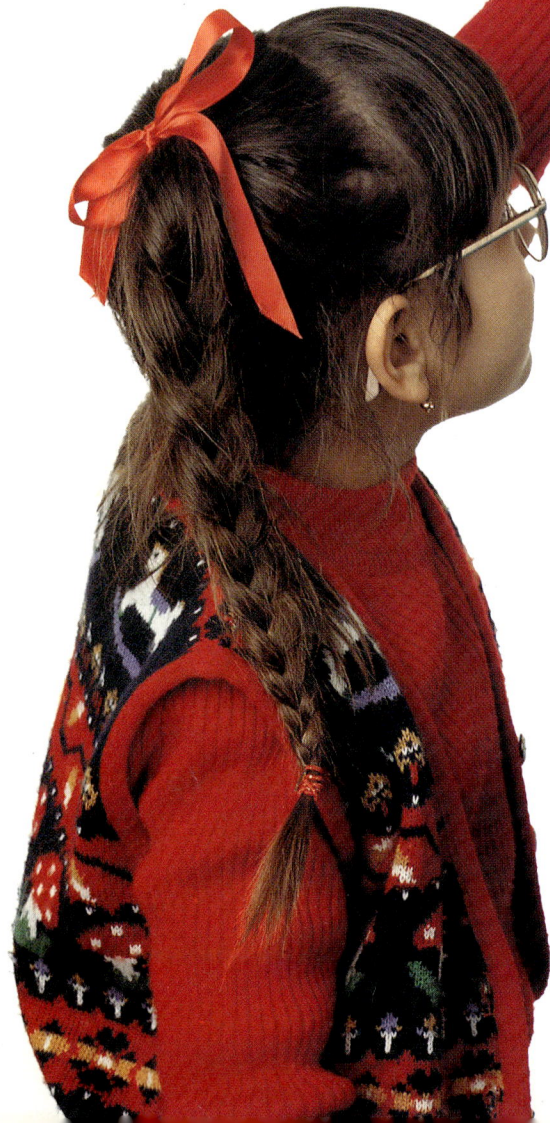

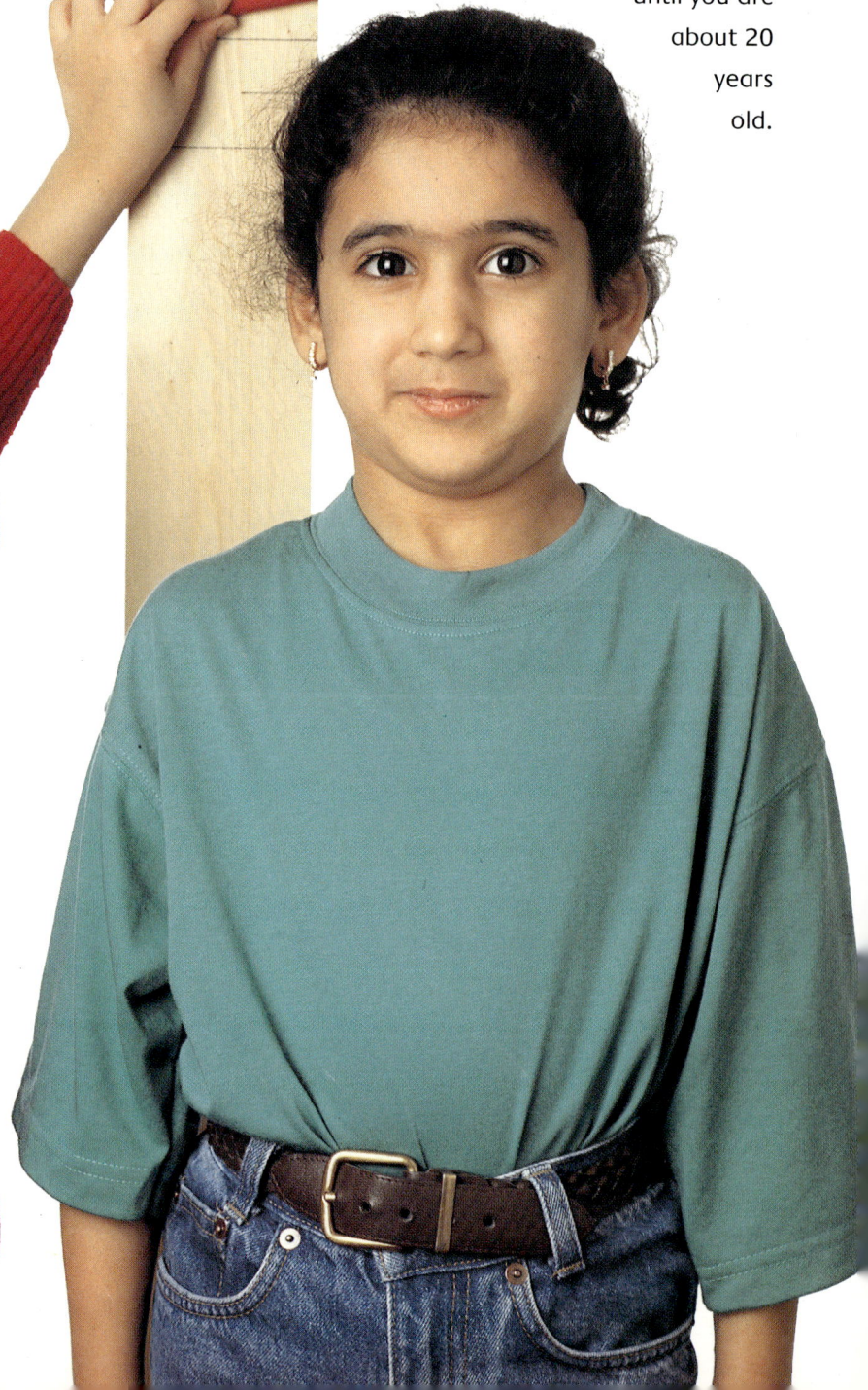

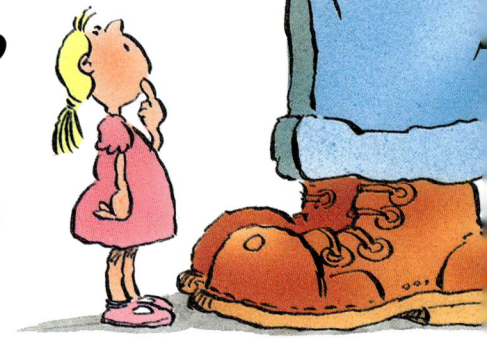

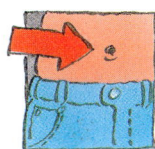

What is my tummy button?

When you were growing inside your mum's tummy, you were joined to her through a special tube. Your tummy button is the place where this tube went into your body. Through this tube, you got food and air from your mother. When you were born, the tube was cut and it shrivelled up to become your tummy button. You didn't need the tube because you started to breathe and feed on your own.

The tube which joins a baby to its mother is about 50 centimetres long.

tube called umbilical cord linking baby to mother

eight-month-old baby floating in bag of liquid

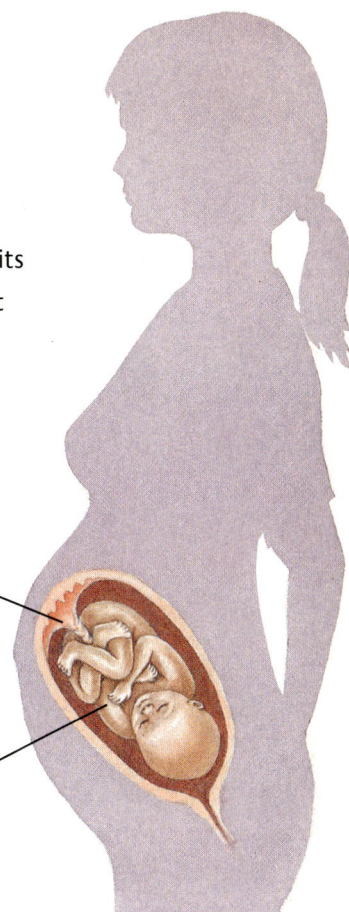

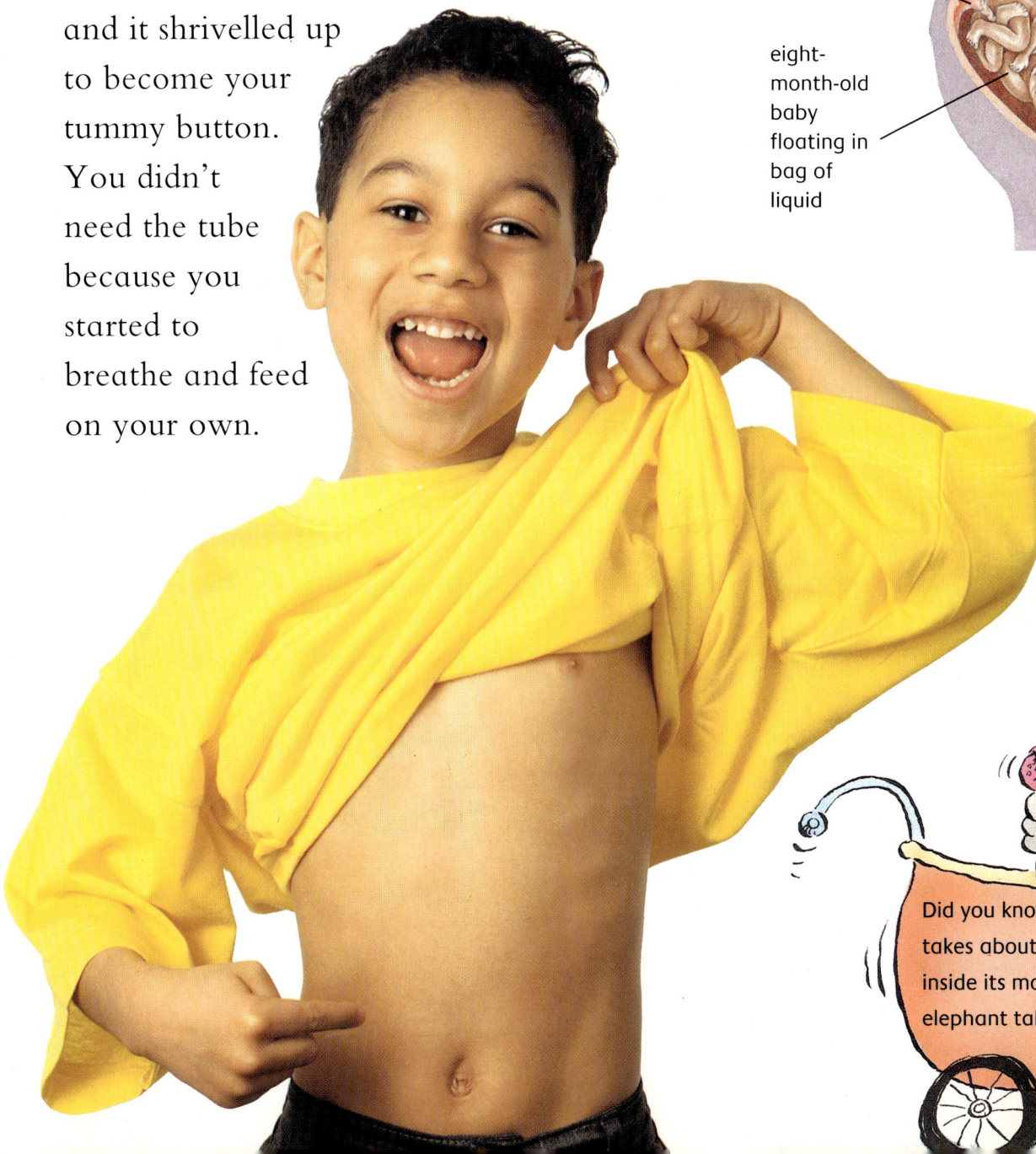

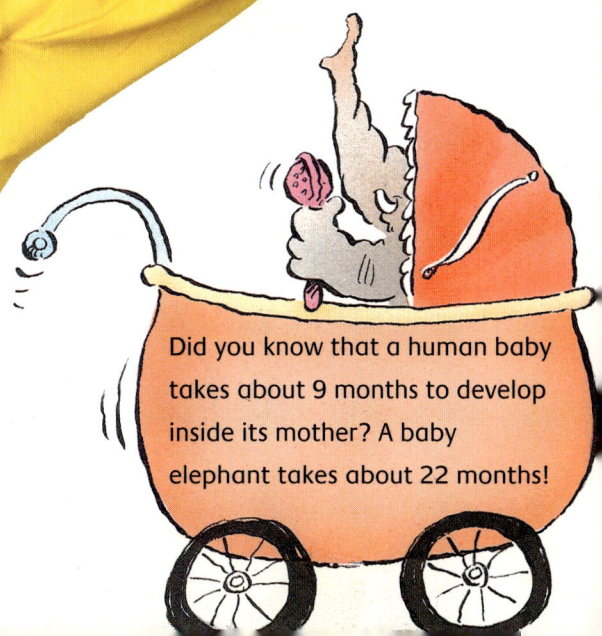

Did you know that a human baby takes about 9 months to develop inside its mother? A baby elephant takes about 22 months!

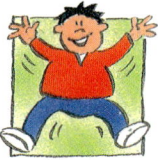

More about your body

Can you jump and stretch like this? So that you can jump, breathe, see, hear, eat and grow, all the different parts of your body have to work together. Even though everyone looks a bit different, our bodies all have the same basic parts inside and work in the same way.

You use your **eyes**, **ears**, **nose**, **tongue** and **skin** to sense what is happening around you.

Inside your head, your **brain** is in charge of your whole body. It collects information from inside and outside your body, makes sense of the information and tells your body what to do.

Before you were born, you grew inside your mum's tummy. You were joined to her at the place where your tummy button is now.

Your **skin** is a tough, waterproof coating which protects your whole body and keeps it clean.

Your **bones** support and protect your whole body. **Muscles** pull bones into different positions so you can move about.

Inside your chest, your **heart** pumps blood through **blood vessels** which go all over your body.

You breathe air into your **lungs** in your chest. You need air as it helps you to speak and to get energy from your food.

Your **teeth**, **stomach** and **intestines** break down food into smaller and smaller pieces so your body can use it. This is called **digestion**.

A chemical code of instructions called **genes** controls what your body is like inside and outside. You inherit half your genes from your mother and half from your father.

Genes are inside the microscopic building blocks called **cells** which your body is made of. There are 50 million million cells in your body.

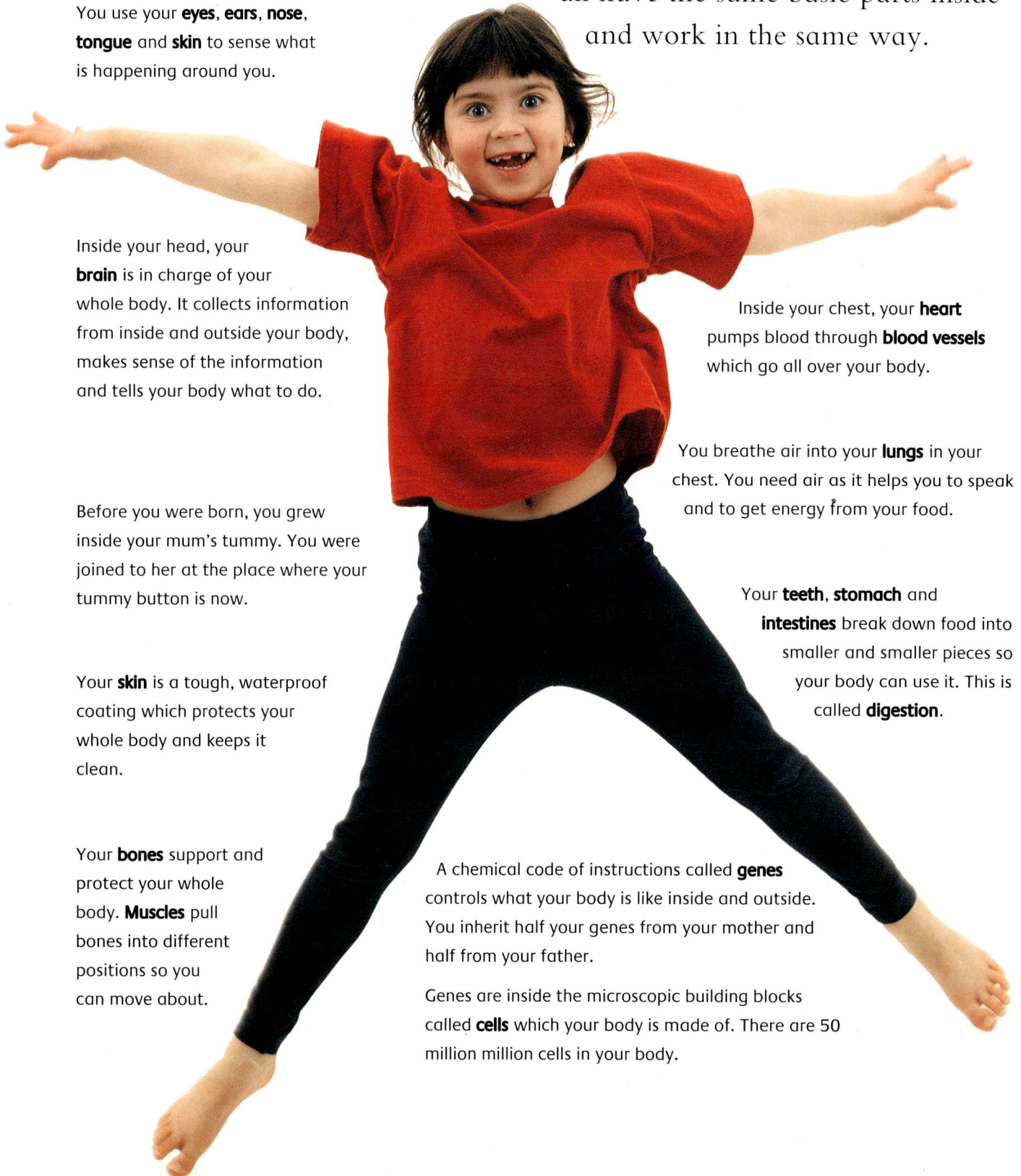

Here are some names of different parts of your body, and what they mean.

Hair follicle A little pocket in the skin from which hair grows – the root of a hair.

Pupil The hole in each eye which opens in the dark to let extra light into the eye.

Blood vessels
Tubes which carry food, oxygen and wastes around the body. Arteries carry blood to the heart and veins carry blood away from the heart. The smallest tubes, called capillaries, go all over the body.

Heart A strong and special muscle in the middle of your chest, which pumps blood around your body.

Liver A complex chemical factory involved in digestion, cleaning the blood and storing nutrients.

Intestines Long tubes in the abdomen where food is broken down so that goodness and energy can be taken into the body.

Skeleton
A framework of bones which touch at joints and are held together by strong bands called ligaments.

Melanin The brown dye which gives skin, hair and eyes some of their colour

Oesophagus A tube behind the trachea leading from the throat to the stomach.

Trachea or windpipe. Tube from the throat to the lungs.

Lungs Large bags in the chest where a gas in the air – oxygen – is taken into the blood and another gas – carbon dioxide – goes back into the air.

Diaphragm A sheet of muscle under your lungs used for breathing.

Stomach A stretchy bag where food is broken up.

Bladder A stretchy bag which stores waste fluids until you are ready to go to the toilet.

Femur
The thigh bone – the longest and strongest bone in the body.

Muscles
Stretchy, elastic materials which are joined onto bones. They can get shorter and longer to pull bones into different positions.

Epidermis The outer layer of the skin.

Keratin The tough substance which nails and hair are made of.

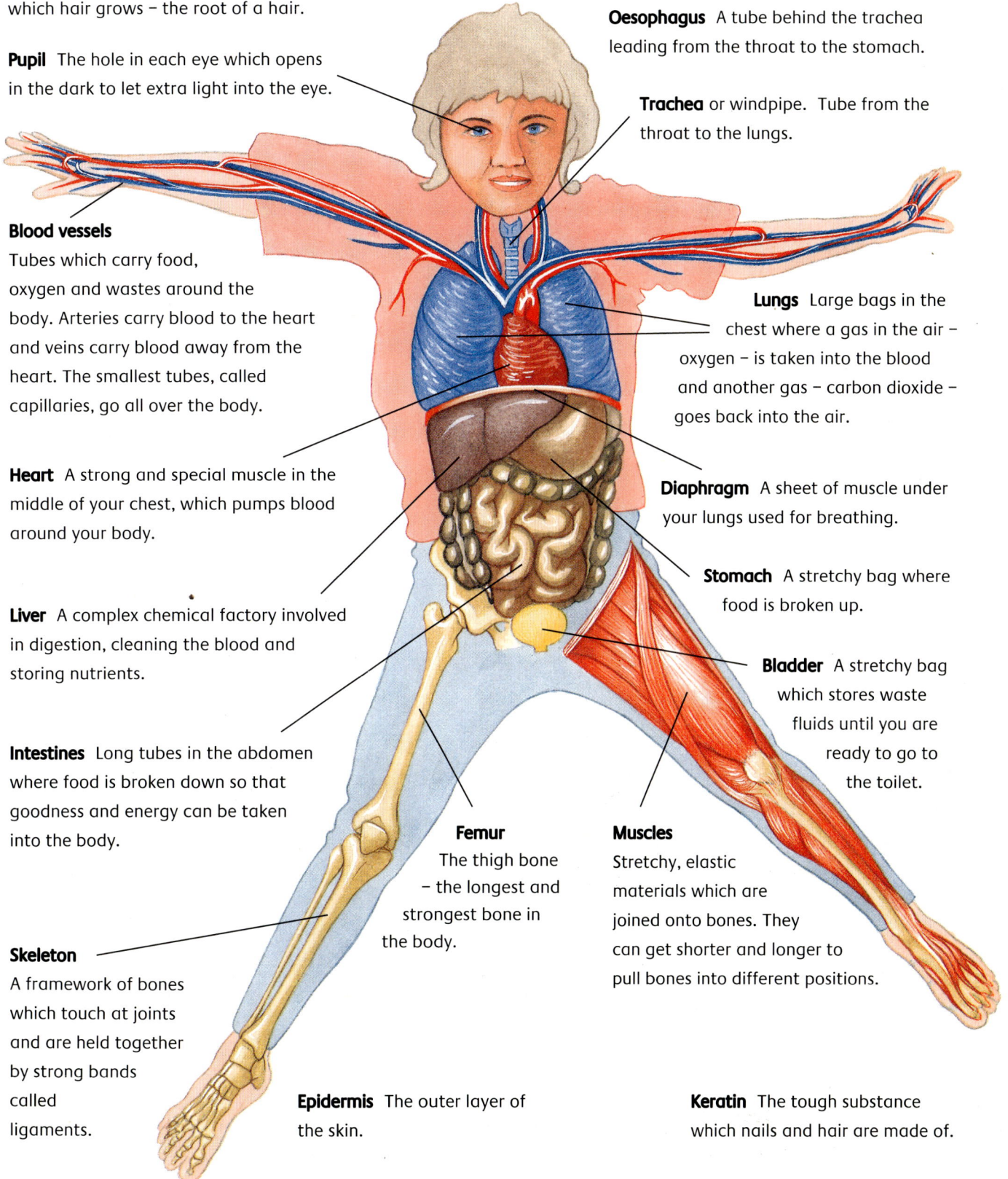

Answers to quizzes

Page

7 **1 a** You have about 5 million hairs on your whole body; **2 c**; **3 d**. Fingernails grow four times faster than toenails.

9 **1** False. People sleep for about one third of their life; **2** True; **3** True; **4** False. *Stegosaurus* was as long as three small cars but its brain was only the size of a walnut. It was probably the most stupid dinosaur. **5** True. We don't usually remember all our dreams, often only the last one.

11 **1** True; **2** True; **3** False. Crickets have ears on their knees; **4** True; **5** False. Tears are made all the time, day or night, whether you are happy or sad.

17 **1** False. An apple only gives you enough energy to swim for about 5 minutes; **2** True; **3** True; **4** False. A cow has one stomach with 4 chambers in it. **5** True.

25 **1** False. A mouse's heart beats up to 600 times a minute. **2** True; **3** True; **4** True.

27 **1** False. Too much fatty food makes you put on weight and can cause heart problems; **2** True; **3** True; **4** False. Children need more sleep than adults because they have a lot of growing to do and new experiences to think about.

Index

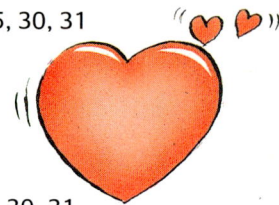

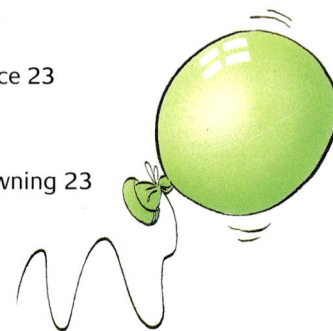